BBQ R

70 Of The Best Ever Barbecue Vegetarian Recipes...Revealed!

Samantha Michaels

Table of Contents

Samantha Michaels

Publishers Notes

Disclaimer

This publication is intended to provide helpful and informative material. It is not intended to diagnose, treat, cure, or prevent any health problem or condition, nor is intended to replace the advice of a physician. No action should be taken solely on the contents of this book. Always consult your physician or qualified health-care professional on any matters regarding your health and before adopting any suggestions in this book or drawing inferences from it.

The author and publisher specifically disclaim all responsibility for any liability, loss or risk, personal or otherwise, which is incurred as a consequence, directly or indirectly, from the use or application of any contents of this book.

Any and all product names referenced within this book are the trademarks of their respective owners. None of these owners have sponsored, authorized, endorsed, or approved this book.

Always read all information provided by the manufacturers' product labels before using their products. The author and publisher are not responsible for claims made by manufacturers.

© **2013**

Manufactured in the United States of America

ENJOY YOUR FREE DOWNLOADS?

PLEASE CLICK HERE TO GIVE ME SOME REVIEWS ON THE BOOK ...APPRECIATE IT!!

MORE 70 BEST EVER RECIPES EBOOKS REVEALED AT MY AUTHOR PAGE:-

CLICK HERE TO ACCESS THEM NOW

Introduction

Would you like to ensure that any vegetarians who come to a barbecue have as wonderful time as the rest of your guests? Well you can by making sure that you prepare the right kinds of foods for them.

Although vegetarians can eat whatever they want most choose not to. But they shouldn't feel as if they are a second-class citizen because of this. When preparing the food for a barbecue to which such people have been invited it is important to find out what sort of vegetarian they are. This will then help you to plan your barbecue much better.

In order to help you with planning the menu for your next barbecue to which vegetarians have been invited we take a brief look below at what types there are.

Type 1 – Pescatarian (Pescetarian)

These types of vegetarians are the ones that will choose not to eat any king of meat or animal flesh other than fish. Although the term isn't used very often there are many people who are choosing to adopt this type of vegetarian diet. Normally they do so because of health issues or before they decide to move on to becoming a fully-fledged vegetarian.

Type 2 – Semi Vegetarian (Flexitarian)

This is the kind of person who chooses to mainly follow a vegetarian diet, but will occasionally choose to eat meat as well.

Type 3 – Vegetarian

Most people when they hear the term vegetarian will of course think of someone who doesn't eat animal flesh of any kind including fish. However these people do continue to eat eggs and dairy products. In fact what these people are referred to, as is being a lacto ovo vegetarian. There may however be some people at your barbecue who are lacto vegetarians, meaning that they will continue to include dairy products in their diet but not eggs. Whereas those known only as a ovo vegetarian will of course continue to eat eggs but will exclude dairy products from their diet.

Type 4 – Vegan

This is the strictest of all diets that vegetarians will follow. These are the kind of people who will not eat any kind of meat or fish and will not consume eggs or dairy products. Furthermore they won't eat any processed foods because they are likely to contain ingredients derived from animals.

Type 5 – Raw Vegan

Such people will only eat foods that have been unprocessed meaning that they haven't been heated above 115 degrees Fahrenheit. The people who follow this particular diet believe that when food has been cooked above this temperature it loses a large amount of the nutrients contained within it and so is harmful to their bodies.

Type 6 – Macrobiotic

This is considered by some to be the healthiest of all vegetarian diets one can follow. It requires the eating of unprocessed vegan foods such as fruits, vegetables and whole grains. However unlike some of the other vegetarian diets mentioned above it does allow the follower to eat fish occasionally. They do however avoid the consumption of sugars and refined oils. Also when following this diet there is a lot of emphasis placed on the eating of Asian vegetables such as sea vegetables (seaweed) and daikon.

Chapter 1 – Vegetable Barbecue Recipes

Recipe 1 – Spicy Grilled Corn on the Cob Recipe

There are numerous ways in which corn on the cob can be cooked on the barbecue. However this particular helps to give a kick to what can sometimes be quite a bland tasting food.

Ingredients

4 Corn On The Cob
½ Teaspoon Lemon Juice Per Ear Of Corn
¼ Teaspoon Cayenne Pepper Per Ear Of Corn
¼ Teaspoon Chilli Powder Per Ear Of Corn
¼ Teaspoon Salt Per Ear Of Corn

Instructions

1. Get the barbecue started making sure that you place the grill 6 inches above the heat source, as you want to cook the corn on a medium heat.

2. Once the barbecue has heated up place the corn on the grill and cook until the corn starts to char and you can insert the tip of a knife easily into a kernel.

3. After removing from the heat drizzle each ear of corn with lemon juice before then sprinkling the cayenne pepper, chilli powder and salt over them. Then serve to your guests.

Recipe 2 – Smoked Corn on the Cob

To make this particular recipe you will first need to soak each cob of corn in water for a few hours whilst still in their husks. Once the corn has finished soaking rub with olive oil and green onions before placing them on the barbecue to cook for an hour so. It is important that at no stage do you remove the corn from the husks.

Ingredients

6 to 12 Ears Of Corn With Husks Still Intact
60ml Olive Oil
1 Bunch Green Onions Finely Chopped

Instructions

1. Gently pull the husks of the corn back without removing them completely. Then remove any silk from inside. Once this has been done place the husks back around the corn.

2. Now take each piece of corn and place in large pan of water ensuring that they fully covered by it and leave there for a few hours.

3. About 20 minutes before you intend to remove the corn from the water get the barbecue fired up. Remember to add some woodchips to the barbecue to help smoke the corn when you place it on the barbecue.

4. After removing the corn from the water gently pull back the husks again and then rub over the olive oil and green onions and place the husks back around the corn. Now place on the barbecue and close the lid. Leave the corn to cook for between 1 and 1 ½ hours.

5. As soon as the corn is ready remove from the barbecue and serve to your guests. Let them pull back the husks and enjoy the aromas that are released.

Recipe 3 – Grilled Sweet Potatoes with Peaches

If you are looking to present your vegetarian guests with something a little more unusual then this is a recipe you may want to try.

Ingredients

4 Sweet Potatoes
2 Peaches Sliced
825ml Vegetarian Baked Beans

75grams Onions Diced
Salt And Pepper To Taste

Instructions

1. Wash the sweet potatoes and pierce the skin several times with the point of a knife. Then place the papers on a paper towel before placing them in a microwave and cooking them on high for 10 minutes or until they become soft.

2. Take eight pieces of heavy weight aluminum foil that have been cut into 12-inch squares. On to this place a half of a sweet potato from which some of the flesh inside has been removed in order to make a narrow space.

3. Now in a bowl combine together the baked beans, slices of peach, onion and the sweet potato you scooped out from the skins earlier. Add some salt and pepper to season before then placing this mixture equally in to each of the potato halves.

4. Once you have filled up each potato bring up the sides of the foil and seal. Make sure that you leave some space between the top of the potato and the point where the foil is sealed to allow steam to have room to expand whilst the potatoes are cooking.

5. Now place the potato parcels on the grill, which has been positioned 4 inches above the heat source. Cook them for around 20 minutes, which will be sufficient time for the food inside to become warmed through. Then serve to your guests still in the foil when cooked.

Recipe 4 – Grilled Chilli Oil Potatoes

This is a very simple dish to prepare and can be served as a main for any vegetarian guests you have invited to your barbecue or as a side dish to those who will be eating meat or fish.

Ingredients

900 to 1300 grams Red Potatoes Cut Into 1 Inch Cubes
1 Red Bell Pepper Cut Into Strips

1 Small Onion Chopped
2 Tablespoons Olive Oil
2 Teaspoons Chilli Powder
1 Teaspoon Salt
½ Teaspoon Garlic Powder
¼ Teaspoon Red Pepper Flakes

Aluminum Foil

Instructions

1. Preheat the barbecue and place the grill 6 inches above the heat source as you will want to cook the potatoes on a medium heat.

2. Whilst the barbecue is heating up into a bowl combine together the potato cubes, strips of pepper, onion, olive oil, chilli powder, salt, garlic powder and pepper flakes. Stir well to ensure that the potatoes are covered well in all the other ingredients.

3. Take too large pieces of aluminum foil and place one on top of the other. Now take the potato mixture and place in the center and then fold the sides of the aluminum foil up to create a parcel. Don't seal the parcels too tightly because some steam will form inside whilst the potatoes are cooking.

4. Now place the parcel on to the barbecue and cook them for 15 minutes. Then turn the parcels before then cooking for a further 15 to 18 minutes before then serving to your guests.

5. After removing from barbecue cut open the parcel with a pair of kitchen scissors and leave to stand for a couple of minutes before then removing them from the foil and serving to your guests.

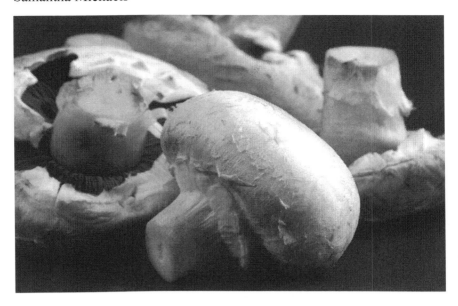

Recipe 5 – Mushroom Burger

Even though this is a dish designed to be enjoyed by vegetarians many of us who eat meat will enjoy this dish as well. The reason being that mushrooms not only seem to taste a bit like meat when cooked but have a similar texture to meat when cooked. The inclusion of pinto beans in this burger also helps to provide lots of protein and fiber.

Ingredients

177grams Fresh Mushrooms Diced
425gram Can Pinto Beans
1 Onion Diced
3 Green Onions Diced
1 Garlic Clove Minced
½ Teaspoon Cumin
2 Tablespoons Vegetable Oil
1 Teaspoon Parsley
Salt And Pepper To Taste

Instructions

1. Take the onions and garlic and sauté them in a frying pan for 3 to 5 minutes or until the onions have become soft. Then to this add the green onions, cumin and diced mushrooms and cook for a further 5 minutes or until the mushrooms are cooked. Now set to one side.

2. In a food processor place the beans and turn on until they have formed a kind of mash. If you don't have a food processor then you can use a fork or potato masher instead.

3. Once the beans have been mashed place this mixture into a bowl and to this add the mushroom mixture along with the parsley. Plus add some salt and pepper to taste. Stir all the ingredients together until they are well combined.

4. Now shape equal amounts of this mixture into patties and place in the refrigerator for a short while before then placing inside a fish basket and cooking on a medium heat on the barbecue for about 3 minutes on each side. Once cooked serve to your guests in a whole wheat bun.

Recipe 6 – Black Bean Burgers

As well as these types of vegetarian burgers being easy to make they also taste very nice as well. When cooking them on the barbecue it is best if you place them inside a fish basket.

Ingredients

½ Onion Diced
1 Can Black Beans Well Drained
118grams Flour
2 Slices Bread Crumbled
1 Teaspoon Garlic Powder
1 Teaspoon Onion Powder
½ Teaspoon Seasoned Salt
Salt And Pepper To Taste

Instructions

1. In a frying place the diced onion with some vegetable and cook for about 3 to 5 minutes or until the onions have become soft. Set to one side to cool a little.

2. Now into a large bowl place the beans and mash with a fork or potato masher until they are almost smooth. Then to this add the onions and also the flour, bread crumbs, garlic power, onion powder and seasoned salt. When adding the flour do so a small amount at the time and make sure it is combined well before adding any more with the other ingredients.

3. Once all the ingredients have been combined together now divide it into equal amounts and form burger patties from them. Ideally the patties you should make be about ¼ inch thick. Then place in the refrigerator for about 20 minutes before then placing on a preheated barbecue and cook until the patties have become firm.

If you want the best way to cook these burgers on a barbecue is to place them in a fish basket. Not only does it help them to retain their shape better, but also turning them over is a lot easier.

Recipe 7 – Vegetable Veggie Burgers

This is a burger that contains a great deal of fiber and is also extremely healthy. You may even find some of your meat eating guests wants to try these out because they smell and taste so delicious when cooked.

Ingredients

118grams Corn Kernels
7 Mushrooms Diced
3 Green Onions Diced
½ Red Bell Pepper Diced
1 Carrot Grated
1 Small Potato Grated
2 Garlic Cloves Minced
1 Teaspoon Cumin
3 Tablespoons Olive Oil
60grams Soft (Silken) Tofu

118grams Bread Crumbs
Salt And Pepper To Taste

Instructions

1. In food processor place the tofu and process until it has become creamy in texture. Remove from processor and place to one side for use later.

2. Now into a frying pan and place the diced mushrooms, corn kernels, green onions and bell pepper with 1 tablespoon of olive oil and cook for 3 to 5 minutes. Then to this add the garlic and cumin and cook for a further one minute. Then remove from the heat.

3. Once the above ingredients have cooled slightly to this add the carrot, potato and tofu along with some salt and pepper. Then start to add to this mixture the bread crumbs. You may find that you don't need all the breadcrumbs to help ensure that the other ingredients used hold together.

4. Once all the ingredients are combined and are holding together divide up into equal amounts and form into patties. Place on a clean plate, cover and place in the refrigerator for at least an hour.

5. Now take the remaining oil and brush over the barbecue grill before placing the veggie burgers on it. Cook each burger for about 6 minutes not forgetting to turn them half way through the cooking time. Then serve to your guests in a whole wheat bun or alongside a fresh crisp green salad.

Recipe 8 – Barbecued Stuffed Acorn Squash

This dish may not seem to contain very many ingredients but it does provide your vegetarian guests with a very hearty meal. If you are having problems finding Acorn Squash you can use a butternut squash instead.

Ingredients

3 Acorn Squash
790gram Can Of Vegetarian Baked Beans

4 Tablespoons Barbecue Sauce

2 Tablespoons Maple Syrup

4 Tablespoons Dark Brown Sugar

3 Tablespoons Butter Or Margarine

240grams Hickory Wood Chips Soaked In Water For 1 Hour Before Then Being Drained

Instructions

1. Take each squash and cut in half along its width. Then slice around ¼ inch off the rounded end of the squash so that they are able to sit upright. Now scrap all the seeds out using a spoon and throw away.

2. Now into a bowl place the baked beans, barbecue sauce, maple syrup and brown sugar and mix well together. Once this is done you divide the mixture into six equal portions and place one portion into each half of the squash. Then top each with ½ tablespoon of butter or margarine.

3. Next turn on the barbecue and place the grill at least 6 inches above the heat source. If you are using a charcoal barbecue to cook the food on then the soaked wood chips can be placed directly on to the charcoal just before cooking of the squash begins. However if you are using a gas barbecue the wood chips need to be placed in either a smoke box or pouch. Also you mustn't start cooking the squash on your gas barbecue until the box or pouch starts to produce smoke.

4. Once the barbecue is ready place the squash on the grill, which you can lightly oil first to prevent them from sticking and close the lid. Leave the squash to cook until the feel soft to the touch and the filling inside each one has turned brown in color and is starting to bubble. You will find that the squash will need about an hour to cook. As soon as the squash is cooked serve to your guests immediately.

Recipe 9 – Grilled Stuffed Chilli Rellenos or Green Bell Peppers

This particular recipe is suitable not only for vegetarians but also vegans. To make it suitable for vegans to eat simply omit the cheese from the recipe.

Ingredients

6 Large Poblano Chillies or Green Bell Peppers
2 Tablespoons Olive Oil
1 Medium Onion Finely Chopped
2 Garlic Cloves Finely Chopped
2 Jalapeno Chillies Seeded And Chopped
½ Red Bell Pepper Finely Chopped
118grams Freshly Chopped Cilantro
1 Teaspoon Ground Cumin
793gram Can Vegetarian Baked Beans Drained
1 to 3 Teaspoons Hot Sauce To Taste
340grams Pepper Jack Or Monterey Jack Cheese Coarsely Grated
Salt To Taste
Freshly Ground Black Pepper To Taste

Instructions

1. Cut the Poblano chillies or bell peppers in half lengthwise. Then scrape out all the seeds so a space is made for the filling to sit in.

2. In a frying pan place two tablespoons of olive oil and to this add the onion, garlic, jalapeno chillies, bell pepper, cilantro and cumin and cook over a medium heat for about 4 minutes or until the onions have turned golden brown.

3. Now remove the pan from the heat and very slowly stir in the baked beans, hot sauce and 226grams of the cheese. Then add salt and pepper to taste. Once this has been done spoon equal amounts of the mixture into the chillies or peppers and then sprinkles the remaining cheese over the top.

4. Next place the chillies or peppers on the grill, which has been placed 6 inches above the heat source and cook on a medium heat

for around 30 to 40 minutes. By the end of this cooking time the chillies or peppers should have become tender and the cheese will have gone brown and the filling inside will start to bubble. As soon as they are ready remove from barbecue and serve to your guests with some rice or couscous.

Recipe 10 – Portobello Mushroom Burgers

Not only will your vegetarian guests enjoy these burgers so will many of your others. The great thing about these particular burgers is that they don't take very long to prepare or to cook.

Ingredients

4 Portobello Mushroom Caps
60ml Balsamic Vinegar
2 Tablespoons Olive Oil
1 Teaspoon Dried Basil
1 Teaspoon Dried Oregano
1 Tablespoon Garlic Minced
Salt And Pepper To Taste
4 X 25gram Slices Provolone Cheese

Instructions

1. Place the mushroom caps in a shallow dish smooth side up. Then into a small bowl place the balsamic vinegar, dried basil and oregano, salt and pepper and whisk well together. Now pour this mixture over the mushroom caps and leave to stand for 15 minutes at room temperature. It is important that whilst the mushrooms are marinating in the mixture that you turn them over twice.

2. Whilst the mushrooms are marinating in the balsamic vinegar you should get the barbecue going ready to then cook them when the 15 minutes marinating time is up. Place the grill of the barbecue between 4 and 6 inches above the heat source, as you want to cook the mushrooms on a medium to high heat.

3. As soon as the barbecue is heated up lightly brush the grill with some oil before then placing the mushrooms on it. Any marinade left over in the dish should be used to baste the mushrooms whilst

they are cooking. Grill each mushroom for 5 to 8 minutes on each side or until they become tender. As well as brushing them with the remaining marinade often you should top the mushrooms the slices of cheese during the last two minutes of cooking. Also place the cheese on the mushrooms when the underside is showing.

4. Once the mushrooms are cooked either serve alone on in a toasted whole wheat roll.

Recipe 11 – Grilled Asparagus

A very quick and easy dish to prepare that could either be served as a main course or as a side dish to all your guests.

Ingredients

450grams Fresh Asparagus Spears Trimmed
1 Tablespoon Olive Oil
Salt And Pepper To Taste

Instructions

1. Preheat the barbecue and place the grill as close to the heat source as possible as you will be cooking these on a very high heat for a very short space of time.

2. Now take the trimmed asparagus spears and lightly coat them with the olive oil and sprinkle with some salt and freshly ground black pepper. Then place on the grill and cook for between 2 and 3 minutes or until they become tender.

3. Once cooked place on a clean plate and serve to your guests alone or with other delicious vegetarian barbecue recipes contained in this book.

Recipe 12 – Grilled Portobello Mushrooms

These types of Portobello mushrooms are simple to prepare and to cook. Yet even so they offer something a little different to your vegetarian guests.

Samantha Michaels

Ingredients

3 Portobello Mushrooms
60ml Canola Oil
3 Tablespoons Onion Chopped
4 Garlic Cloves Minced
4 Tablespoons Balsamic Vinegar

Instructions

1. Clean the mushrooms and remove the stems, which can then be used in some other dish later. Once clean place the mushrooms in a shallow dish with the gills facing upwards.

2. Next into a small bowl place the canola oil, chopped onion, minced garlic and balsamic vinegar and whisk until combined together well. Then pour of this mixture evenly over the mushrooms and leave them to marinate it in for at least 1 hour.

3. Once the barbecue is hot enough you need to cook them on a high heat for 10 minutes. During this time turn them over occasionally to ensure that they are cooked right through. Once they are cooked serve immediately to your guests with some salad and new potatoes.

Recipe 13 – Foil Wrapped Veggies

As well as being a meal that you could serve on their own they make a wonderful accompaniment to other food you may be serving at your barbecue.

Ingredients

1.1kg New Potatoes Thinly Sliced
1 Large Sweet Potato Thinly Sliced
2 Vidalia Onions Cut Into ¼ Thick Slices
220grams Fresh Green Beans Cut Into 1 Inch Pieces
1 Sprig Fresh Rosemary
1 Sprig Fresh Thyme
2 Tablespoons Olive Oil
Salt And Freshly Ground Black Pepper To Taste

60ml Olive Oil

Instructions

1. Whilst preparing the vegetables you should be getting the barbecue going so it is as hot as possible for when the vegetables need to be cooked. Make sure that the grill is a close to the heat source as possible because you want to cook these parcels on as high a heat as possible.

2. After the vegetables have been prepared place them in a large bowl and to them add the rosemary and thyme as well as 2 tablespoons of olive oil. Plus don't forget to sprinkle in some salt and pepper to taste.

3. Now take 2 or 3 sheets of aluminum foil and place one on top of the other. You will need a total of around 12 sheets of foil in all to make up the parcels containing the vegetables. On the top layer of foil brush with some more olive oil before then distribute the vegetables evenly between each.

4. Seal each parcel up by gathering the sides above the vegetable mixture. However don't seal the parcels too tightly as steam will be produced whilst the vegetables are cooking.

5. Once the parcels are sealed place on the preheated barbecue and cook for around 30 minutes. It is important that during this time you turn the parcels at least once to ensure that all the ingredients inside are cooked evenly. Serve to your guests once the potatoes have become tender still in the aluminum foil but with the top cut open.

Recipe 14 – Eggplant Mixed Grill

A great dish that you may find all your guests would like more of even though it is very simple to prepare and cook.

Ingredients

1 Red Onion Cut Into Wedges
18 Spears Fresh Asparagus Trimmed

12 Crimini Mushrooms Cleaned And Stems Removed
1 (450gram) Eggplant Sliced Into ¼ Inch Rounds
1 Red Bell Pepper Seeded And Cut Into Wedges
1 Yellow Bell Pepper Seeded And Cut Into Wedges
2 Tablespoons Olive Oil
2 Tablespoons Fresh Parsley Chopped
2 Tablespoons Fresh Oregano Chopped
2 Tablespoons Fresh Basil Chopped
1 Tablespoon Balsamic Vinegar
1 Teaspoon Salt
½ Teaspoon Freshly Ground Black Pepper
6 Garlic Cloves Minced

Instructions

1. In a large bowl combine together the olive oil, fresh parsley, oregano, basil, balsamic vinegar, salt, black pepper and garlic. Then pour into a large resealable bag. Then into this place all the eggplant slices, wedges of red and yellow pepper, asparagus spears, mushrooms and onion wedges.

2. Seal the bag and turn over several times to ensure that all the vegetables have been coated in the marinade. Now place the bag in the refrigerator and leave there for 2 hours. It is important that whilst the vegetables are marinating in the sauce that you turn the bag over occasionally to ensure that all sides of the vegetables are coated in the marinade.

3. When the barbecue is heated up lightly oil the grill before then removing the vegetables from the bag and placing them on the barbecue. Cook these vegetables for 12 minutes. Half way through this time make sure that you turn the vegetables over to ensure that they are cooked through evenly. As soon as the vegetables are tender place on a clean plate and serve them to your hungry guests.

Recipe 15 – Grilled Yellow Squash

This is a very simple recipe but is sure to be something that delights all guests at your barbecue.

Ingredients

4 Medium Sized Yellow Squash
120ml Extra Virgin Olive Oil
2 Garlic Cloves Crushed
Salt And Freshly Ground Black Pepper To Taste

Instructions

1. Start the barbecue up and place the grill 6 inches above heat source, as you will be cooking the squash on a medium heat.

2. Now whilst the barbecue is heating up cut the squash horizontally into ¼ to ½ inch thick slices. Cutting to this size will actually prevent the slices from falling through the grill.

3. Next take the olive and to this add the crushed garlic cloves and cook on a medium heat until the garlic begins to sizzle and the oil becomes fragrant. Remove from heat and then brush this mixture over the slices of squash and sprinkle over them some salt and pepper.

4. Now take the slices of squash and place on the barbecue and cook for 5 to 10 minutes on each side or until they become tender. Make sure that whilst cooking the yellow squash you brush them regularly with any leftover garlic oil to prevent them from burning or sticking to the barbecue grill.

5. Once the squash is cooked place on a clean plate and serve to your guests with some rice or couscous or some pita bread.

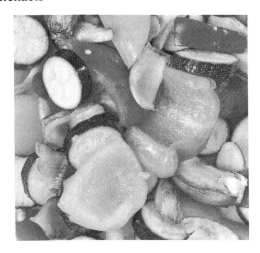

Recipe 16 – Marinated Barbecued Vegetables

The marinade in which you leave and then cook the vegetables helps to bring out even more of their wonderful flavors.

Ingredients

1 Small Eggplant Cut Into ¾ Inch Thick Slices
2 Small Red Bell Peppers Seeded And Cut Into Wide Strips
3 Zucchini Sliced
6 Fresh Mushrooms Stems Removed
60ml Olive Oil
60ml Lemon Juice
60gram Fresh Basil Chopped
2 Garlic Gloves Peeled And Minced

Instructions

1. Into a medium sized bowl place the slices of eggplant, strips of pepper, slices of zucchini and mushrooms.

2. Now into another bowl place the olive oil, lemon juice, basil and garlic and whisk together well before then pouring over the vegetables. Cover the bowl with vegetables over and place in the refrigerator allow them to marinate in the olive oil mixture for at least 1 hour.

3. About 20 minutes before you remove the vegetables from refrigerator get the barbecue started. Remember to place the grill of the barbecue 4 inches above the heat source, as you will want to cook the marinated vegetables on a high heat.

4. After removing the vegetables from the marinade place them directly on to the grill or thread them onto skewers. Then cook them over a high heat for about 4 to 6 minutes. When cooking make sure that you turn the vegetables over half way through the cooking time to ensure that they are cooked properly. Also to help prevent them from sticking or burning you should regularly baste them with any of the left over marinade.

5. Once the vegetables are all cooked place on a clean plate and serve to your guests.

Recipe 17 – Grilled Tequila Portobello Mushrooms

Although Portobello mushrooms taste wonderful on their own the inclusion of tequila helps to add a little extra to this amazing vegetable.

Ingredients

1 Large Portobello Mushroom Cut Into ¾ Inch Slices
60ml Tequila
35grams Unsalted Butter Melted
2 Tablespoons Roasted Garlic Oil
Juice Of 1 Lime
3 Garlic Cloves Minced

Instructions

1. In a small bowl combine together the tequila, butter, garlic oil, lime juice and minced garlic. Once all these have been combined leave to stand for at least 15 minutes.

2. In fact whilst this mixture is being left to stand you should now be lighting or turning on the barbecue ready for when you want to start cooking.

3. Once the barbecue has heated up enough lightly brush some oil over the grate. Then you should lightly brush the mushroom slices with the tequila mixture made earlier before then placing them on to the grill to cook.

4. You should cook the mushroom slices until they start to wilt, then they need to be turned over. Once turned over brush some more of the tequila mixture over the slices of mushroom for a minute or so more or until the mushrooms have become tender. You will need to watch carefully when cooking the mushrooms as there is a risk of them burning if left on the barbecue for too long.

Recipe 18 – Grilled Zucchini and Summer Squash Parcels

These are two vegetables that you will find plenty of available fresh in your local supermarket; greengrocers or farmers market through the summer time. However this is also a great dish to prepare later in the year.

Ingredients

2 Zucchini Cut In Half Lengthwise Then Into ¼ Inch Thick Slices
1 Summer Squash Thinly Sliced
170grams Butter
1 Tablespoon Salt
2 Tablespoons Freshly Ground Black Pepper
2 Tablespoons Garlic Powder

Instructions

1. It is important that you start the barbecue going before you start preparing the ingredients to make this dish. This will help to ensure that the barbecue has reached the right temperature for cooking the parcels at. Also make sure that the grill on the barbecue is placed 4 to 6 inches above the heat source, as you will want to cook these parcels on a medium to high heat.

2. Whilst the barbecue is heating up take a large piece of aluminum foil and onto it place the slices of zucchini and summer squash. Then dot them with the butter and sprinkle over them all the salt, freshly ground black pepper and garlic powder.

3. Now bring up the sides of the aluminum foil so that the vegetables you have placed on it are sealed inside. Now place this parcel on to the barbecue grill and allow to remain on there for at least 20 minutes or until the squash and zucchini inside have become tender.

4. Once the vegetables are cooked remove from foil and place on to plates served with some fresh natural yogurt, pitta bread or some rice.

Recipe 19 – Asian Inspired Grilled Asparagus

Although you may want to serve this dish to your guests hot, it tastes just as wonderful when served cold. Plus of course this dish doesn't take a great deal to prepare or cook so can be served to unscheduled guests who are vegetarians in a matter of minutes.

Ingredients

1 Bunch Of Fresh Asparagus Trimmed
1 Tablespoon Soy Sauce
1 Tablespoon Sesame Oil

Instructions

1. After trimming the asparagus place them on a lightly oiled barbecue grill that is set for cooking them on a medium to high heat.

2. Now cook the asparagus until they have turned bright green and they have grill marks on them. This should take around 10 minutes and it is important half way through this time that you turn the asparagus over to ensure that it is cooked through evenly.

3. Once cooked transfer to a serving bowl or plate and leave to one side too cool for a little while.

4. Whilst the asparagus is cooling into a small bowl place the soy sauce and sesame oil and whisk until they are combined well together. Then pour this mixture over the asparagus before then

covering and placing in the refrigerator. Leave them in the refrigerator for at least 30 minutes before then serving.

Recipe 20 – Grilled Baked Potatoes

Fed up with eating baked potatoes as you would normally, where you add some butter to them. Well give this recipe a try and you may never want to eat baked potatoes like it any more.

Ingredients

4 Large Baking Potatoes Cut Into Quarters
2 Tablespoons Olive Oil
2 Teaspoons Freshly Ground Black Pepper
2 Teaspoons Garlic Powder
2 Teaspoons Dried Rosemary
Salt To Taste

Instructions

1. Place the potatoes in a large pot and cover them with water. Now bring the water to the boil and then cook the potatoes over a medium to high heat for 10 minutes or just as the potatoes start to become tender.

2. Whilst the potatoes are cooking it is a good idea to get the barbecue started so by the time you remove the potatoes from the water it will be ready for them to cook on it. Place the grill of the barbecue 4 to 6 inches above heat source remember you will be cooking these on a medium to high heat.

3. After removing the potatoes from the water now place them in a bowl and into the pour the olive oil and sprinkle in the black pepper, rosemary and salt. Toss the potatoes very gently to make sure that all quarters are covered in the oil mixture and them place each quarter on to the barbecue skin side down.

4. Now leave them to cook on the barbecue for about 15 minutes then remove from it and place on clean plate. Before serving any leftover oil should be drizzled over the potatoes.

Chapter 2 – Tofu Barbecue Recipes

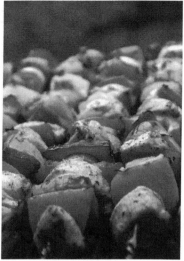

Recipe 1 – Tofu Kebabs with a Mustard Mayonnaise Dressing

Not only will those who are vegetarian enjoy eating these kebabs so will the non vegetarians when you serve them at your next barbecue.

Ingredients

250gram Regular Tofu Drained And Pressed
150ml Mayonnaise
1 Tablespoon Dijon Mustard
1 Tablespoon Medium Curry Paste
1 Garlic Clove Crushed
1 Inch Piece Fresh Ginger Peeled And Grated
Salt And Freshly Ground Black Pepper
16 Cherry Tomatoes
8 Shallots Halved
16 Button Mushrooms
1 Tablespoon Smooth Mango Chutney

Instructions

1. Cut the tofu into bite size pieces and then place these in a shallow dish. Now set to one side whilst you make the marinade.

2. To make the marinade place the mayonnaise in a bowl with the Dijon mustard, curry paste, garlic and ginger. Stir well together then season with some salt and pepper. Once all these ingredients have been combined together now pour the mixture over the pieces of tofu and stir everything around very gently. This will help to ensure that all sides of the tofu are coated in the marinade. Cover the dish with some cling film and then leave for 30 minutes.

3. Whilst the tofu is marinating in the sauce you can now get the barbecue ready for cooking the kebabs.

4. After the marinating time is over start to thread the pieces of tofu on to wooden skewers that have been soaking in water along with the tomatoes, shallots and button mushrooms. Keep any marinade left over for serving with the kebabs later.

5. Just before you place the kebabs onto the barbecue make sure that you brush the grill with some vegetable oil to prevent them from sticking to it.

6. You should cook the kebabs until the marinade starts to bubble and the vegetables and tofu start to turn a golden brown.

7. Whilst the kebabs are cooking place the remaining marinade in a small saucepan and gently heat through. Add to this the tablespoon of smooth mango chutney.

8. Once the kebabs are cooked place on a bed of plain rice and then drizzle over the marinade sauce in the saucepan.

Recipe 2 – Tofu and Green Onion Veggie Burgers

As well as being very tasty these particular burgers are also very nutritious because of the inclusion of wheat germ in them. Not only is this recipe suitable for vegetarians but also for vegans.

Ingredients

½ Container Firm Or Extra Firm Tofu Mashed
1 Onion Diced
3 Green Onions Diced
2 Tablespoon Wheat Germ
2 Tablespoon Flour
2 Tablespoon Garlic Powder
2 Tablespoon Soy Sauce
Dash Freshly Ground Black Pepper

Instructions

1. In a large bowl place the tofu, onions, wheat germ, flour, garlic powder, soy sauce and black pepper and mix well together.

2. Once all the ingredients have been combined together divide up into equal amounts and form into patties. Then leave them in the refrigerator for about 30 minutes.

3. Whilst the patties are resting in the refrigerator get the barbecue going. Make sure that you place the grill six inches above the heat source, as you want to cook these on a medium heat to prevent them from burning or drying out.

4. If you want to avoid the hassle of trying to turn each burger over as you cook them on the barbecue then place them inside a fish basket. Cook for around 10 minutes (5 minutes on each side) until the outsides of them are brown and crispy. Then serve to your guests with a whole wheat roll and some salad.

Recipe 3 – Devilled Tofu Kebabs

This particular recipe helps to add some spice to an ingredient that looks very bland and unappealing to eat.

Ingredients

300gram Firm Smoked Tofu Cut Into Cubes
8 Shallots Or Button Onions
8 Small New Potatoes
2 Tablespoons Tomato Puree
2 Tablespoons Light Soy Sauce

1 Tablespoon Sunflower Oil
1 Tablespoon Clear Honey
1 Tablespoon Wholegrain Mustard
1 Courgette Peeled And Sliced
1 Red Pepper Deseeded And Diced

Instructions

1. In a small bowl place the shallots or button onions and over them pour boiling water then put to onside for 5 minutes.

2. Into a saucepan of water place the potatoes and cook these for at least 7 minutes until they are tender. Once cooked remove from water and pat dry.

3. Next into another bowl place the tomato puree, soy sauce, sunflower oil, honey, wholegrain mustard and season with salt and pepper. Mix all these ingredients well together before then adding the cubes of tofu to them. Mix again to ensure that all the tofu is then covered in the sauce. Cover the bowl over and leave the tofu to marinate for at least 10 minutes.

4. Whilst the tofu is marinating get the barbecue going ready for when you make the kebabs. As the barbecue is heating up you can now start to make the kebabs. First remove the shallots (button onions) from the water and peel them. Then cook them in boiling water for 3 minutes. Drain and set to one side for the moment.

5. Now take some skewers (if using wooden ones make sure that these have been soaked in water for at least 30 minutes). On to each skewer thread cubes of tofu followed by a shallot, potato, a slice of courgette and a piece of pepper. The amount of ingredients used in this recipe will make you 8 kebabs.

6. Once all the kebabs are ready now lightly oil the grill and then place the kebabs on it. Grill each kebab on the barbecue for 10 minutes making sure that you turn them over frequently to prevent them not only from sticking to the grill but also to prevent them burning. Any left over marinade should be brushed over the kebabs as they cook.

Once cooked serve the kebabs either with some plain rice or with a pita bread.

Recipe 4 – Grilled Tofu with Mediterranean Chopped Salad

Tofu has quite a mild flavor and will benefit from you using quite an intense lemon and garlic based marinade. If at all possible allow the tofu to marinate in the garlic and lemon for at least 8 hours to help it absorb as much of their flavors as possible.

Ingredients

400grams Extra Firm Tofu (Water Packed Variety)
60ml Fresh Lemon Juice
1 Tablespoon Extra Virgin Olive Oil
3 Garlic Cloves Minced
2 Tablespoons Dried Oregano
½ Teaspoon Salt To Taste
Freshly Ground Black Pepper To Taste

Mediterranean Chopped Salad

2 Medium Sized Tomatoes Seeded And Diced
230grams Seedless Cucumber Diced
60grams Scallions (Green Onions) Chopped
60grams Fresh Parsley Coarsely Chopped
60grams Kalamata Olives Pitted And Coarsely Chopped
2 Tablespoons Extra Virgin Olive Oil
1 Tablespoon White Wine Vinegar
¼ Teaspoon Salt To Taste
Freshly Ground Black Pepper To Taste

Instructions

1. Whilst the barbecue is heating up in a bowl place the lemon juice, oil, garlic, oregano, salt and bowl and mix well together. Once combined in a small pot place 2 tablespoons of the mixture, as you will use this for basting the tofu later when it is cooking.

2. Next remove the tofu from its packaging and rinse well. Then cut it up into eight slices each measuring around ½ inch thick. Place the slices of tofu into a shallow dish and pour over the marinade made earlier. Make sure that you turn the tofu over to ensure that it is fully covered in the marinade. Now cover the dish and place in the refrigerator for at least 30 minutes. However if at all possible let it remain in the marinade for between 4 and 8 hours.

3. Whilst the tofu is marinating you can now begin making the Mediterranean chopped salad. To do this simply place the tomatoes, cucumber, scallions, parsley, olives, oil, vinegar, salt and pepper into a bowl and toss very gently. Cover and place in the refrigerator whilst the tofu is cooking.

4. To cook the tofu remove from the marinade and place on to the barbecue grill which has been lightly oiled first. Any marinade left over in the dish can now be discarded. When cooking the tofu it should be done over a medium to high heat and each side of it should be cooked for between 3 and 4 minutes. Whilst cooking make sure that you baste it regularly with the marinade you saved earlier.

The best way to make attractive grill marks on the tofu as it cooks is to rotate it 90 degrees halfway through grilling. Doing this will create a cross hatch design on it.

5. As soon as the tofu is cooked and has turned a light brown in color place on plates and top with some of the Mediterranean chopped salad and serve to your guests.

Recipe 5 – Cilantro Lime Grilled Tofu

The cilantro and lime help to give the tofu a little pizzazz.

Ingredients

400grams Firm Tofu
60ml Fresh Lime Juice
1 Tablespoon Olive Oil
75grams Fresh Cilantro Chopped
2 Garlic Cloves Minced

2 Teaspoons Chilli Powder
¼ Teaspoon Cayenne Pepper
Salt And Freshly Ground Black Pepper To Taste

Instructions

1. After removing the tofu from its packaging place on a plate and on top place another plate on to which at least 5lbs of weight has been placed. Leave the tofu between the two plates for between 20 and 30 minutes as this will help to remove some if not all of the liquid in the tofu. Any liquid that comes out of the tofu should be drained off and discarded.

2. Now cut the tofu lengthwise into 4 thick slices or if you want to cook it on skewers then cut it into ¼ thick cubes. Then place the sliced or cubed tofu on to a plate.

3. Next you need to make the marinade for the tofu. In to a bowl place the lime juice, chopped cilantro, garlic, chilli powder and cayenne pepper and whisk together. Halfway through whisking these ingredients together add some salt and pepper to taste.

4. Normally you would pour any marinade you make over the tofu, however with this one you must brush it on, remembering to do all sides of the tofu. Now cover the plate on which the tofu is with some cling film and then place in the refrigerator for at least 2 hours. However if you want more of the marinade flavors to be absorbed by the tofu then it is best to leave it in the marinade overnight.

5. About 20 minutes before you remove the tofu from the refrigerator you should get your barbecue going. Place the grill on which the tofu is to be cooked 6 inches above the heat source to ensure that it with be cooked on a medium heat.

6. Once the barbecue is hot enough before placing the tofu on to the grill lightly brush some vegetable oil over it. Any leftover marinade should not be discarded but can be brushed over the tofu whilst it is cooking. Cook the tofu for a total of 10 to 15 minutes or until black spots start to appear on it. Also do not forget

to turn the tofu over occasionally as this will help to ensure that it is cooked right through.

7. As soon as the tofu is cooked place on a clean plate and serve to your guests.

Recipe 6 – Grilled Tofu and Sautéed Asian Greens

The sweet and sour flavours used in the marinade help to make tofu, which is a bland sort of food, come alive.

Ingredients

400grams Firm Tofu Drained
60ml Low Sodium Soy Sauce
1 Teaspoon Asian Sesame Oil
1 ½ Teaspoons Packed Dark Brown Sugar
1 ½ Teaspoons Fresh Ginger Peeled And Finely Grated
1 Small Garlic Clove Minced
¼ Teaspoon Tabasco Sauce Or Dried Hot Red Pepper Flakes
1 Tablespoon + 1 Teaspoon Vegetable Oil
2 x 140gram Bags Of Asian Greens Or Baby Spinach

Instructions

1. Cut the tofu crosswise into 6 slices and then arrange on a triple layer of paper towels and then on top of this place a baking sheet or baking pan and leave to stand for 2 minutes. After this time remove the paper from above and below and replace with more dry paper towels. Repeat this process twice more.

2. Whilst you are attempting to drain as much liquid from the tofu as possible you can now make the marinade. Into a bowl place the soy sauce, sesame oil, brown sugar, ginger, garlic, Tabasco sauce or red pepper flakes and a tablespoon of vegetable oil and mix well together. Now pour into a shallow dish and to this add the slices of tofu and leave to marinate in the mixture for 8 minutes. It is important that whilst the tofu is marinating in the sauce you turn it over every couple of minutes. This will help to ensure that as much of the marinade is absorbed by the tofu.

3. Whilst the tofu is marinating in the sauce you can start the barbecue up. Cook it on a medium heat making sure that you turn it over once during the cooking time. To ensure that the tofu is cooked correctly it should remain on the grill for between 4 and 6 minutes.

4. Whilst the tofu is cooking on the barbecue you now need to prepare the Asian greens or baby spinach to go with it. Take the other tablespoon of oil and place in a frying pan or skillet and once it has heated up you add the greens and toss them until they start to wilt. Any left over marinade can then be poured over the greens.

5. Once the greens and tofu are cooked then take the greens out of the frying pan letting any excess marinade to drip off first and then place equal amounts on to two plates. Then on top of this place three slices of the cooked tofu and serve to your vegetarian guests.

Recipe 7 – Spicy Grilled Tofu

If you want to avoid the tofu sticking to the barbecue when cooking then make sure that you remove as much water from it as possible. Plus also you use extra firm tofu whenever possible.

Ingredients

450grams Extra Firm Tofu Drained Cut Lengthwise Into 8 Slices
120ml Fresh Lime Juice
80ml Maple Syrup
60ml Low Sodium Tamari Or Soy Sauce
2 Teaspoons Chilli Paste With Garlic
3 Garlic Cloves Minced
¼ Teaspoon Freshly Ground Black Pepper

Instructions

1. After slicing up the tofu place on several layers of paper towel and cover with several more. Then leave to stand for 20 minutes. Occasionally place some weight on to the paper towels as this will help to squeeze even more water out.

2. After the 20 minutes have elapsed remove the tofu from between the paper towels and place in a shallow baking dish. Ready for marinade that you are about to make to be poured over them.

3. To make the marinade in a small bowl place the lime juice, maple syrup, Tamari or soy sauce, chilli paste, minced garlic and pepper and whisk. Then pour over the tofu making sure that you turn the tofu over so it is coated all over in the sauce. Then cover very lightly with some plastic wrap before then placing in the refrigerator to marinate. 4 hours is sufficient for marinating the tofu in the sauce. But if you want more of the sauces flavors to be absorbed by the tofu then leave it to marinate in it overnight.

4. Just before you place the tofu on the barbecue to cook, make sure that you have brushed the grill with oil and it has been placed six inches above the heat source, as you want to cook the tofu on a medium heat. Any marinade left over after you remove the tofu from the dish should be kept for use later.

5. Cook the tofu on each side for between 3 and 4 minutes or until they outside has started to go brown and crisp. Once cooked remove from barbecue then place back in the dish with the remaining marinade toss lightly and then serve to your guests.

Recipe 8 – Tofu and Eggplant Hobo Bundles

If you invite guests to your barbecue who don't eat meat then preparing these for them means you don't actually have to worry about what they are eating coming into contact with what your other guests are going to be enjoying.

Ingredients

560grams Firm Tofu Cut Into 16 Pieces
340grams Asian Eggplant Quartered Lengthwise And Cut Into Pieces
2 Tablespoons Minced Garlic
2 Tablespoons Minced Ginger
60ml Reduced Sodium Soy Sauce
5 Tablespoons Vegetable Oil

2 Green Onions Chopped

Instructions

1. Place the pieces of tofu and eggplant into a resealable bag with the minced garlic, ginger, soy sauce, vegetable oil and onions and seal. Then shake the bag very gently to ensure that all the ingredients are combined together well and the eggplant and tofu are covered in the sauce. Place in the refrigerator and leave there for at least an hour.

2. Once the barbecue has heated up divide the eggplant and tofu mixture up between 4 large sheets of aluminum foil. Fold the sides of the aluminum foil up and secure. Then place the bundles onto the barbecue grill and cook for 10 minutes. It is important that halfway through the cooking time you turn the bundles over once to make sure all inside is cooked through evenly.

3. Remove from barbecue and cut open the bundles before then placing on plates to serve to your guests. Best served with a rice salad.

Recipe 9 – Grilled Vegetable and Tofu Salad

A very simple dish to prepare but if you want to ensure that as much of the flavor of the marinade is absorbed by the tofu and vegetables you should leave them to marinate in the sauce overnight.

Ingredients

450grams Firm Tofu Drained
180ml Italian Salad Dressing
340grams Yellow Summer Squash Cut Lengthwise Then Cut Into 2 Inch Pieces
2 Large Orange And/Or Red Sweet Peppers Seeded And Quartered
Hot Peppers Seeded (You Can Use As Many As You Want0
120grams Quinoa
120grams Quick Cooking Barley
120grams Shredded Sorrel Or Spinach

Instructions

1. Take the tofu and cut lengthwise in to 8 slices, which should be around ½ inch thick and place these into a shallow baking dish. Pour over 60ml of the Italian salad dressing before then covering the dish with some plastic wrap and leave to one side.

2. Next take all the vegetables and place these into a large resealable bag that you then place in deep bowl. Over these pour 3 tablespoons of the dressing and close the bag before turning it over several times to make sure all the vegetables have been coated with the dressing. Place both the vegetables and tofu into the fridge along with the remaining dress and leave there for at least 4 hours.

3. Just before you start cooking the vegetables and tofu remove them from the dressing and discard any that remains. You should first place the vegetables on to the grill and cook these for between 6 and 8 minutes or until they are tender. Do not forget to turn them over half way through the cooking time to prevent them from burning.

4. Two minutes after you have placed the vegetables on the barbecue you can now place the tofu on. Just like the vegetables the tofu should be cooked over a medium heat and for around 4 to 6 minutes. Again making sure to turn them over once half way through cooking.

5. Once the tofu is cooked (should now be light brown in color) remove from barbecue and cut in half diagonally to form triangles. Then place to one side for serving shortly.

6. After removing the vegetables from the barbecue place in a bowl and pour over the remaining dressing and toss them very lightly to coat the vegetables with it.

7. Just before you place the tofu and vegetables on to the barbecue you should be preparing the quinoa and the barley. After rinsing place the quinoa and barley into a pan of boiling water and simmer on a low heat for 15 minutes or until most of the water has been absorbed. Drain and then add to them the shredded sorrel. Place

equal amounts of this mixture on to a plate before then topping with slices of tofu and grilled vegetables.

Recipe 10 – Tofu and Pepper Kebabs

This particular recipe is not suitable if you have guests who happen to suffer from a nut allergy.

Ingredients

255grams Firm Tofu Drained And Cut Into Small Cubes
50grams Dry Roasted Peanuts
2 Red Bell Peppers
2 Green Bell Peppers Seeded And Cut Into Large Chunks

Instructions

1. Take the dry roasted peanuts and place in a blender or food processor and turn on the machine and grind the peanuts down to form pieces similar to breadcrumbs. Pour these then on to a plate.

2. Whilst the barbecue is heating up take four large skewers and on to these thread pieces of tofu, and pieces of red and green bell peppers. Place to one side until the barbecue has heated up.

3. Once the barbecue has heated up grill the kebabs for 10 minutes, remembering to turn them over after 5 minutes. Plus don't forget to oil the surface of the grill before placing the kebabs on it to prevent them from sticking.

4. After the kebabs are cooked through remove barbecue place on a plate and sprinkle over the ground dry roasted peanuts. Serve them with any kind of dipping sauce. Would highly recommend using a sweet chilli dipping sauce with these kebabs.

Recipe 11 – Grilled Lime Tofu with Lime Mayonnaise

The acidity of the lime helps to cut through the blandness of the tofu.

Ingredients

Samantha Michaels

450gram Block Firm Or Extra Firm Tofu Drained
1 Garlic Clove Minced
25grams Fresh Ginger Peeled And Grated
Freshly Ground Black Pepper To Taste
Salt To Taste
1 Tablespoon Sesame Seed Oil
Juice Of 2 Limes (Use Zest In Lime Mayonnaise)

Lime Mayonnaise

120ml Mayonnaise
Juice From 1 Large Lime
Zest From 2 Other Limes
Teaspoon Sugar
Pinch Salt

Instructions

1. After draining the tofu well slice it into 6 or 8 pieces and then place into a resealable plastic bag. Now add into the bag the lime juice, garlic, ginger and the sesame seed oil. Seal the bag up and turn it over several times to ensure all the pieces of tofu are coated in the sauce. Place in the refrigerator and leave the tofu to marinate in the sauce for at least 8 hours. However if possible it is best to leave the tofu to marinate over night.

2. Once the barbecue has heated up remove the tofu from the bag and pat dry with some paper towels. Sprinkle over some salt and pepper and place then on to the lightly oiled barbecue grill. The grill itself should be set 4 inches above the heat source, as you want to cook the tofu over a high heat. Cook on each side for about 5 minutes or until it starts to turn brown.

3. Whilst the tofu is cooking you can prepare the lime mayonnaise to go with it. Simply place the mayonnaise, lime juice and lime zest into a bowl and stir gently with a spoon.

4. As soon as the tofu is cooked placed on to plates and beside the slices of tofu place a spoonful of the mayonnaise and serve to your guests.

Recipe 12 – Tomato, Onion and Tofu Kebabs

These kebabs are very refreshing and would be great served with some couscous along with a mint yogurt dip.

Ingredients

450grams Extra Firm Water Packed Tofu Drained
1 Tablespoon Lime Juice
2 Tablespoons Low Sodium Soy Sauce
1 Teaspoon Fresh Ginger Root Minced
1 Teaspoon Sriracha Sauce
16 Fresh Mint Leaves
12 Cherry Tomatoes
1 Onion Peeled Quartered And Separated Into Layers
60ml Hoisin Sauce

Instructions

1. Cut the tofu into 1 ½ inch squares and place on a towel and then place another towel on top on to which a heavy weight of some kind must be placed. Leave like this for 15 minutes so more of the water in the tofu can be removed.

2. Whilst the tofu is being pressed take a bowl and into this place the lime juice, soy sauce, ginger and sriracha sauce and mix well. Set to one side to use shortly.

3. After pressing the tofu take the pieces and place in the sauce you made earlier remembering to stir it well so that all pieces of the tofu are coated in the mixture. Cover the bowl over and place in the refrigerator and leave the tofu to marinate in the mixture for 30 minutes or longer.

4. Next take the wooden skewers and place in a bowl of water to soak, as this will then prevent them from burning when placed on the barbecue.

5. Once the allotted time for the tofu to marinate has passed remove from the refrigerator and start to assemble the kebabs. On to each skewer place one piece of tofu, one piece of onion, one

cherry tomato and one mint leaf. Do this until all of the skewers have been used.

6. The barbecue should have been preheated to a high heat and when ready place the kebabs on it after lightly oiling the grill and cook for 10 minutes. When cooking the kebabs make sure that you turn them occasionally to prevent them from burning and to ensure that they are cooked right through.

7. After 10 minutes of cooking brush over the kebabs the hoisin sauce and cook them for a further 5 minutes, remember to turn them occasionally and cook until the vegetables have softened and the tofu is well glazed. Then serve on plates with the couscous and mint yogurt dip.

Recipe 13 – Cajun Grilled Tofu

This particular recipe takes tofu to a whole new level. As well as being low in fat and carbs this dish is high in protein and makes a very flavorsome main course for the non meat eaters at your barbecue.

Ingredients

450grams Extra Firm Tofu Drained
120ml Canola Oil
2 Tablespoons Cajun Seasoning Rub

Cajun Seasoning Rub Ingredients

3 Tablespoons Salt
1 ½ Teaspoons Sweet Paprika
1 Tablespoon Onion Powder
1 Tablespoon Cayenne Powder
½ Teaspoon White Pepper
2 Teaspoons Dried Thyme
½ Teaspoon Freshly Ground Black Pepper
1 Teaspoon Dried Oregano

Instructions

1. The first thing you need to do is make the Cajun seasoning rub. To do this simply place all the above ingredients into a small bowl and stir well to blend them together. Once made you can keep this for up to 6 months as long as you store it in an air tight container.

2. After making the seasoning rub the next thing to do is press as much excess water out of the tofu as possible. Once you have done this you cut the tofu into ¾ inch thick slices and place in a shallow baking dish.

3. Now take the canola oil and to this add the seasoning rub you made earlier and mix well. Then brush this mixture all over the tofu and cover with plastic wrap and place in the refrigerator until you are ready to start cooking. Remember the longer you leave the tofu to marinate in the seasoning rub the more of the amazing flavors will have been absorbed by it.

4. It is important that when cooking the tofu you first lightly oil the barbecue grill before placing the tofu on it to prevent it from sticking. Also place the grill 6 inches above the heat source, as you want to cook on a medium to high heat. Cook for between 10 and 12 minutes remembering to turn it over occasionally to ensure that the tofu is cooked right through and is golden brown in color.

5. Once the tofu is cooked place on clean plates and serve to your guests with a crisp green salad and a yogurt dip.

Recipe 14 – Lemon Achiote Grilled Tofu

If you are having problems sourcing achiote powder locally there are numerous places online where such items can be purchased.

Ingredients

340grams Extra Firm Tofu Cut Into 4 Slabs
2 Tablespoons Achiote Powder
¼ Teaspoon Cayenne Pepper
1 Tablespoon Raw Cane Sugar Or Brown Sugar
3 Medium Garlic Cloves Peeled
2 Big Pinches Of Salt
80ml Fresh Squeezed Lemon Juice

Instructions

1. Take the 3 peeled garlic cloves and sprinkle over some salt. Then with the flat side of the blade of a knife press down on the garlic cloves until a paste is formed. Then in to a bowl place the garlic paste, achiote powder, cayenne pepper, brown sugar and lemon juice and whisk well to ensure all these ingredients are combined together.

2. Next take the slabs of tofu and place these in a shallow baking dish and pour the achiote marinade over them. Remember to flip the slabs of tofu over a couple of times to ensure that they are coated all over in the marinade. Plus use your hands to also rub the marinade into the tofu. Now cover the dish with some plastic wrap and place in a refrigerator for at least 1 hour. Whilst the tofu is marinating make sure that you go back a couple of times to turn it over.

3. About 15 minutes before you remove the tofu from the refrigerator you should get the barbecue started. Place the grill 6 inches above the heat source, as you will want to cook the tofu on a medium heat. Once the barbecue is heated up lightly oil the grill before you place the tofu on it.

4. After placing the tofu on the barbecue brush it with any of the remaining marinade and cook for between 10 and 12 minutes, remembering to turn it over occasionally. If you want to create a cross hatch effect on the tofu then as you turn it over rotate it 90 degrees.

5. Once the tofu has turned a golden brown remove and serve either on a crisp green salad or in a whole wheat bun with all the trimmings to your guests.

Recipe 15 – Grilled Tofu Satay

This particular recipe like the others in this book helps to give the tofu a little extra kick. But be careful and do not serve to any of your guests who may have any kind of nut allergy.

Ingredients

900grams Extra Firm Tofu Drained Cut Into 1 Inch Cubes
1 Red Bell Pepper Seeded Cut Into 1 Inch Squares

Marinade

2 Tablespoons Soy Sauce
2 Tablespoons Sesame Oil
2 Tablespoons Sherry

Satay Sauce

180ml Coconut Milk
120ml Natural Style Peanut Butter (Smooth Or Chunky)
2 Garlic Cloves Minced
1 ½ Teaspoons Curry Powder
1 ½ Tablespoons Brown Sugar
1 Tablespoon Lime Juice
1 Tablespoon Canola Oil
1 ½ Tablespoons Soy Sauce
Dash Cayenne Pepper

Instructions

1. In a bowl combine together the soy sauce, sesame oil and sherry to make the marinade. Then to this add the tofu and red pepper and toss gently until they are evenly coated in the marinade. Cover the bowl over with some plastic wrap and place in the refrigerator for between 30 minutes and 8 hours. The longer you leave the tofu to marinate in the sauce the more of its flavor will be absorbed by the tofu.

2. About 20 minutes before you remove the tofu and peppers from the refrigerator get the barbecue started. Whilst the barbecue is heating up you can now make the satay sauce to serve with the tofu.

3. To make the satay sauce place all the ingredients mentioned above in a food processor and blend until a smooth mixture is formed. Remove from processor and place into a serving bowl and set to one side (refrigerate if you wish) ready to use later. However

before setting it aside take about 60ml of the sauce as you will be using this for coating the tofu just before you cook it.

4. To cook the tofu and peppers thread these on to skewers and then brush over them the satay sauce and cook over a high heat for at least 20 minutes. Make sure that you turn the skewers over frequently to prevent the tofu and peppers from burning or until the tofu is cooked through.

5. Allow the kebabs to cool down to room temperature before then serving to your guests along with the remainder of the satay sauce you made earlier.

Recipe 16 – Barbecued Tofu

Adding barbecue sauce to the tofu helps to add a little spice and sweetness to this food.

Ingredients

900grams Medium Firm Tofu Sliced
½ Red Onion Chopped
½ White Onion Chopped
½ Bell Pepper Seeded And Chopped
1 Celery Stick Chopped
2 Tablespoons Olive Oil
4 Garlic Cloves Chopped
Salt To Taste
Pinch Curry Powder
Barbecue Sauce

Instructions

1. Preheat the barbecue placing the grill 6 inches above the heat source, as you will want to cook the tofu on a medium heat.

2. Whilst the barbecue is heating up you can prepare the barbecue sauce for the tofu. To do this place the onions, pepper, celery, olive oil, garlic, salt, curry powder and barbecue sauce in a saucepan and cook over a medium heat for a few minutes. Now set to one side ready to pour over the tofu once it is cooked.

3. Place the tofu on to the lightly oiled barbecue grill and brush over the top some of the barbecue sauce made earlier. Then cook for around 6 minutes before then turning over. Again brush over some of the sauce you made earlier and cook for a further 6 minutes.

4. Once the tofu is cooked place on a clean serving plate and pour over the top the remaining barbecue sauce and serve to your guests.

Recipe 17 – Grilled Tofu and Vegetable Pita Pockets

You may find that many of your meat eating guests will enjoy these as much as your vegetarian ones do. If you have any vegan guests attending your barbecue then remove the feta cheese.

Ingredients

450grams Firm Tofu Drained Cut Into Inch Thick Slices
8 Green Onions
240ml Italian Dressing
3 Tablespoons Fresh Mint Finely Chopped
2 Green Bell Peppers Seeded Quartered Lengthwise
60grams Feta Cheese Crumbled
4 Pita Breads

Instructions

1. Whilst the barbecue is heating up prepare dressing. Simply pour the Italian dressing into a bowl and add the mint. Whisk well into these two ingredients are combined. Then set to one side for use later.

2. Next take the slices of tofu, pepper and the green onions and place on a plate before then brushing over some of the dressing you made earlier. By now the barbecue should be ready and cooking can begin.

3. Take the 4 pita breads and wrap in aluminum foil and place them at the very edge of the barbecue grill to warm through.

4. Next take the slices of tofu, pepper and green onions and place these on the barbecue grill which has been lightly oiled and brush over a little more of the dressing you made earlier. Cook each side of the vegetables for around 4 minutes and each side of the tofu for around 2 to 3 minutes. Once all these are cooked you are now ready to start placing them in the pita breads.

5. Remove the vegetables and tofu from the barbecue and cut the tofu and peppers in ¼ inch pieces. Take the pita breads off the barbecue and make an incision in the top. Now fill each one with pieces of tofu and pepper and top off with 2 of the green onions and sprinkle over a quarter of the crumbled feta cheese. Then drizzle over them the remaining dressing before then serving to your guests.

Recipe 18 – Lemon Herb Grilled Tofu

This recipe is suitable for any vegan guests who may attend your barbecues.

Ingredients

450grams Extra Firm Tofu

Marinade

120ml Olive Oil
80ml Lemon Juice
2 Teaspoons Ground Cumin
2 Teaspoons Dried Oregano
1 Teaspoon Dijon Style Mustard
½ Teaspoon Garlic Salt
1 Teaspoon Lemon Pepper

Instructions

1. After draining the tofu cut into ½ inch slices (cut them slightly thicker if you intend to make the tofu into kebabs). Now place the slices of tofu between some sheets of paper towel and place a weight on top to allow more water to drain out of the tofu. Leave the weight in place for an hour.

2. When the hour has passed remove the weight and take the tofu from inside the paper towels and pat it dry. Then cut the tofu into either triangles or to cubes.

3. Next place the lemon juice, ground cumin, oregano, mustard, garlic salt and lemon pepper in a bowl and whisk until well combined. Then pour into a resealable bag and add to it the tofu and seal. Turn the bag over several times to ensure that the marinade coats all of the tofu and place in the refrigerator for at least 1 hour. If you can leave the tofu to marinate in the sauce for longer then more of the flavor of the sauce will be absorbed by it.

4. Cook the tofu on a medium to high heat on the barbecue for about 10 minutes. Do not forget to turn the tofu over frequently to prevent it from burning. Then serve to your guests with some freshly grilled vegetables or with some green beans, couscous or rice.

Recipe 19 – Harissa Grilled Tofu

Although this is a very simple dish to make to really get the flavor of the marinade running through the tofu it needs to be left in the sauce for sometime. If at all possible make this particular dish up to 3 days before your barbecue is to take place.

Ingredients

450grams Extra Firm Tofu Drained, Pressed, Cut Into 8 Slices
120ml Vegetable Broth
60ml Dry Red Wine
1 Tablespoon Harissa Paste
1 Tablespoon Olive Oil
Juice From ½ Lemon
1 Teaspoon Ground Cumin
½ Teaspoon Fine Sea Salt
Generous Pinch Of Freshly Ground Black Pepper

Optional: Dash Of Liquid Smoke

Instructions

1. Into a bowl place the vegetable broth, red wine, harissa paste, olive oil, lemon juice, ground cumin, sea salt and pepper and whisk well to ensure all ingredients are combined.

2. Now take the slices of tofu and place these in a shallow baking dish and pour over them the marinade you have just made. Remember to turn the slices of tofu over to ensure that they are fully coated in the sauce. Now cover the dish with plastic wrap and place in the refrigerator for up to 3 days.

3. Cook the slices of tofu on a medium to high heat on the barbecue. So the grill should have been placed 4 to 6 inches above the heat source and also make sure that before you place the tofu on the grill it has been brushed with oil. Whilst the tofu is cooking on the barbecue remember to turn it over regularly and also baste with any remaining marinade as well. If you want to create a cross hatch effect on the tofu then rotate it 90 degrees each time you turn it over. Cook the tofu until it has turned golden brown on both sides.

4. Once cooked serve the slices of tofu with some fresh green vegetables and some couscous with onions and corn. Also any left over marinade can then be drizzled over the top to help bring all the elements of the dish together.

Recipe 20 – Grilled Herb Tofu with Avocado Cream

The use of the avocado cream with this dish helps to bring out even more of the wonderful flavors that the tofu has been cooked in. Again a suitable dish to serve to any vegan guests at your barbecue.

Ingredients

340grams Extra Firm Tofu Drained And Patted Dry
2 Tablespoons Extra Virgin Olive Oil
1 Tablespoon Herbs de Provence
¾ Teaspoon Salt
¼ Teaspoon Freshly Ground Black Pepper

Avocado Cream

170grams Ripe Haas Avocado Peeled And Pitted
120grams Fresh Flat Leaf Parsley
120ml Vegetable Broth
80ml Extra Virgin Olive Oil
1 Tablespoon Fresh Lime Juice
1 Garlic Clove Peeled And Smashed
Zest Of 1 Large Lime
Salt And Freshly Ground Black Pepper To Taste

Instructions

1. Cut the tofu in half diagonally to make 2 large triangles then cut each of these into half to make 4 smaller ones. Then cut through each of the smaller triangles horizontally so you end up with 8 tofu triangles. Brush each side of the tofu with the olive oil before then sprinkling over each side the herbs, salt and pepper.

2. Now place on a preheated barbecue and cook for 2 minutes on each side or until they have turned a light golden brown color. Once cooked place on a platter to serve to your guests.

3. To make the cream place the avocado, vegetable broth, flat leaf parsley, olive oil, lime juice and zest and garlic in a food processor and blend until smooth. Then add to this some salt and pepper to taste.

4. Either spoon the cream over the top of the tofu before serving to your guests or place in a bowl beside which your guests can then dip the tofu in.

Chapter 3 – Cheese Barbecue Recipes

Recipe 1 – Halloumi Skewers and Mediterranean Vegetables

Your vegetarian guests will love these skewers especially when served with some warm pitta bread. Plus you will love them, as they are so easy to make.

Ingredients

400grams Halloumi Cheese
1 Garlic Clove Crushed
18 Whole Pitted Black Olives
100ml Olive Oil
3 Large Tomatoes
6 New Potatoes
2 Large Courgettes
1 Red Onion
1 Aubergine
6 Kebab Skewers (If Using Wooden Ones Soak In Water For At Least 30 minutes)
Pitta Bread

Instructions

1. In a food processor blend together the garlic, olives and olive oil to form a kind of marmalade.

2. Cut the Halloumi into 1 inch cubes. Then cut the tomatoes into quarters and remove the seeds and cut the potatoes in half lengthwise. Then boil the potatoes until they are tender then drain. Also cut up the rest of the vegetables in 1 inch cubes.

3. As for the remaining vegetables cut these all into 1 inch cubes ready for threading on to the skewers. On to each skewer alternately thread pieces of Halloumi and vegetables and then pour over them the marmalade you made earlier and leave to marinate in it for at least 2 hours.

4. To cook the kebabs place on the lightly oiled barbecue grill and cook on each side for 2 minutes over a medium to high heat. Whilst the Halloumi and vegetable skewers are cooking wrap the pitta breads in aluminum foil and place at the edge of the barbecue grill to warm through.

5. Just before you remove the skewers from the barbecue remove the pitta breads and place them on plates along with skewers. Then serve to your guests.

Recipe 2 – Halloumi with Saffron Tomato Salad

You can enjoy this salad either as part of a barbecue or just as a light supper. If you intend to have this as a light supper then place the Halloumi in a griddle pan rather than cooking it on the barbecue.

Ingredients

500grams Halloumi Cut Into 1 Inch Chunks
Pinch Saffron Strands
6 Large Red Chilli's Deseeded Cut Into Quarters Lengthwise
200grams Cherry Tomatoes
120ml Extra Virgin Olive Oil
240grams Bulgar Wheat Rinsed
2 Tablespoons Capers Drained And Rinsed
40ml Sherry Vinegar
1 Tablespoon Black Onion Seeds Or Kalonji Seeds
Handful Rocket Leaves

Instructions

1. Light or preheat the barbecue and place 6 to 8 wooden skewers in some warm water for 30 minutes.

2. Whilst the barbecue is heating up place the chunks of Halloumi, strands of saffron, chillis and tomatoes in a bowl with the olive oil. Then season with a little salt and pepper and cover with plastic wrap and leave for 20 minutes.

3. Next take the Bulgar wheat and place it in a bowl before then pouring over boiling water and cover this with plastic wrap and set aside like the Halloumi for 20 minutes. However make sure that you fluff the wheat up occasionally with a fork.

4. Once the barbecue is ready drain of any excess oil from the Halloumi, chillis and tomatoes into a jug and start to thread these ingredients on to the skewers. Then place on to the lightly oiled barbecue grill and cook on each side for 2 minutes.

5. Whilst the kebabs are cooking add to the reserved oil the capers, vinegar and onion seeds and mix well then stir a few spoonfuls of this into the Bulgar wheat before then adding the rocket.

6. Now divide the salad equally among 3 or 4 plates and top off with the kebabs. Then drizzle over the remaining dressing and then serve immediately to your guests.

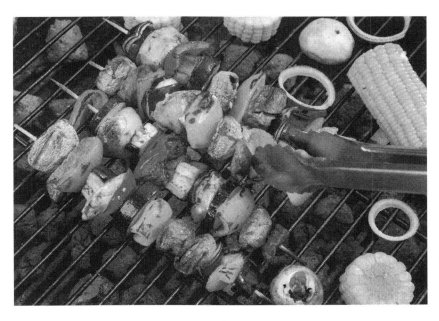

Recipe 3 – Tikka Skewers

No vegetarian at your next barbecue needs to feel left out when you serve up these kebabs to them.

Ingredients

300grams Paneer Cheese Cut Into Chunks
3 Tablespoons Tikka Paste
500grams Yogurt
2 Teaspoon Cumin Seeds
Thumb Size Piece Of Fresh Ginger Peeled And Finely Grated
250gram Small New Potatoes
3 Red Onions Peeled Sliced Into Wedges Through The Root
2 Red Peppers Deseeded And Cut Into Chunks
5 Tablespoon Mango Chutney
1 Small Pack Mint Leaves
250grams Salad Leaves
12 Chapattis

Instructions

1. In a shallow baking dish soak 12 wooden skewers in water for 30 minutes. Whilst the skewers are soaking you can now make the marinade for the kebabs. In a bowl mix together the Tikka paste, 250grams of yogurt, the cumin seeds, grated ginger and season with some salt and pepper. Now set to one side (it is best to keep it in the refrigerator whilst you are preparing the rest of the ingredients to make the kebabs).

2. Next take the small new potatoes and place in a pan of boiling salted water and cook for 7 minutes. Then drain well and allow to cool before then adding these and the cheese to the marinade you made earlier. Make sure that you stir these ingredients around in the marinade well to ensure that they are fully coated in it. Then cover the bowl before then placing back in the refrigerator for at least 2 hours.

3. To assemble the kebabs you simply alternately thread pieces of the marinated cheese and potatoes on to the skewers along with the onions and peppers. Place on a tray and cover until the barbecue has heated up sufficiently.

4. Cook the kebabs on the barbecue whose grill has been lightly oiled for 10 to 15 minutes, making sure you turn them over

occasionally to prevent them from burning, plus also to make sure that they are cooked right through.

5. Whilst the kebabs are on the barbecue prepare the dip and salad, which you will serve with them. To make the dip stir the mango chutney into the other 250grams of yogurt, and to make the salad combine the salad leaves with the mint leaves.

6. A few minutes before you are going to remove the kebabs from the barbecue place the chapattis on it to warm do. Do a few at the time. Then take the kebabs and place them on plates with the chapattis, salad and mango yogurt dip and serve to your guests.

Recipe 4 – Toasty Feta Kebabs

This recipe isn't only very quick and easy to prepare but also is very quick and easy to cook.

Ingredients

200gram Pack Reduce Fat Feta Cheese Cut Into 8 Chunks
½ French Baguette Cut Into Bite Size Chunks
8 Cherry Tomatoes
1 Lemon
Zest Of 1 Lemon
2 Sprigs Fresh Rosemary Chopped
1 Tablespoon Olive Oil

4 Wooden Skewers Soaked In Water For 30 Minutes

Instructions

1. Whilst the barbecue is heating up take the lemon and cut one half of it into wedges and the other half into slices and put to one side.

2. Next take the pieces of bread and thread on to the skewers followed by a piece of feta cheese, a slice of lemon and a tomato. Do this a second time making sure that at the end of each kebab you place one last piece of bread.

3. Just before you begin cooking the kebabs sprinkle over them the lemon zest and rosemary before then drizzling over some olive oil. Grill each kebab on the barbecue for 2 to 4 minutes, making sure that you turn them over. Cook until the feta has turned a golden brown then place on plates along with the lemon wedges.

Recipe 5 – Barbecued Vegetables with Goats Cheese

The sweetness of the vegetables cuts through the acidity of the goat's cheese beautifully.

Ingredients

200grams Firm Goats Cheese
4 Aubergines Cut Into 1 Cm Slices Lengthwise
8 Plum Tomatoes Cut Into 3 Thick Slices Each
2 Bunches Spring Onions Trimmed
150ml Extra Virgin Olive Oil
2 Tablespoons White Wine Vinegar
3 Plump Garlic Cloves Crushed

Large Handful Fresh Basil Leaves

Additional Extra Virgin Olive Oil For Drizzling
8 Flour Tortillas

Instructions

1. Into a large shallow dish place the slices of aubergine, tomatoes and spring onions. Then in a small bowl place the olive oil, white wine vinegar and garlic and mix well add some salt and pepper to season before then pouring over the vegetables. Toss the vegetables very gently to make sure that they are well coated and set to one side whilst you wait for the barbecue to heat up.

2. When the barbecue is heated up remove the aubergines from the marinade and place them on to the lightly oiled barbecue grill and cook for 4 to 5 minutes on each side. Then remove from the barbecue. Next remove the tomatoes and onions from dish and cook these on the barbecue for 3 to 4 minutes, not forgetting to

turn them over half way through the cooking time. Then place them in the same dish as the aubergines.

3. Now take the goats cheese and crumble this over the top of the hot vegetables and then drizzle over some more extra virgin olive oil and toss all of these ingredients together very gently.

4. To serve place the above ingredients on to a clean serving plate and scatter the fresh basil leaves over the top. Don't forget to serve the tortillas warm by placing them on the very edge of barbecue grill for 1 to 2 minutes.

5. Let your guests take one of the tortillas and place a spoonful of the vegetables and cheese into the middle and fold up the tortilla and eat.

Recipe 6 – Roasted Tomato and Feta Parcels

Like other recipes in this book this one allows you to cook food for the meat eating guests at your barbecue at the same time.

Ingredients

200grams Feta Cheese Crumbled
500grams Cherry Tomatoes
Few Sprigs Rosemary
Olive Oil
Balsamic Vinegar

Instructions

1. Take 12 sheets of aluminum foil and place 2 sheets on top of each other to make six parcels into which the cheese and tomatoes can be placed.

2. Now divide the cheese and tomatoes equally between these six sheets of aluminum foil and top of with a sprig of rosemary and drizzle over some olive oil. Then seal the parcels up and place on the barbecue for 10 to 15 minutes or until the tomatoes have begun to burst open and the cheese is soft.

3. As soon as the tomatoes have begun to burst open and the cheese is soft remove the parcels from the barbecue and place on plates and cut the foil open to reveal the food inside. Then drizzle with the balsamic vinegar before then serving to your guests.

Recipe 7 – Falafel and Halloumi Burgers

These burgers are a little unusual but are something that your vegetarian guests will enjoy.

Ingredients

2 X 400grams Tinned Chickpeas Drained
2 Teaspoons Ground Cumin
1 Teaspoon Ground Coriander
2 Green Chillis Chopped
2 Garlic Cloves
½ Small Bunch Spring Onions
1 Teaspoon Salt Flakes
2 Tablespoons Plain Flour
1 Pack Halloumi Diced
Pitta Bread To Serve
Houmous To Serve
Lettuce To Serve
Pickled Chillis To Serve

Instructions

1. To make the burgers place the chickpeas, cumin, coriander, chillis, garlic, spring onions, salt flakes and flour into a food processor and blend. Tip this mixture into a bowl then add to it the diced Halloumi.

2. Now divide up into 6 equal amounts and create 6 burgers. Place these on to a clean plate and put in to the refrigerator to rest whilst the barbecue is heating up.

3. Once the barbecue has heated up remove the burgers from the refrigerator and before placing on the barbecue lightly oil the grill. Then cook each burger for 2 to 3 minutes on each side or until they have turned a golden color.

4. As soon as the burgers are cooked remove from the barbecue and serve with the pitta bread that you have warmed through on the barbecue along with some of the Houmous, lettuce and pickled chillis.

Recipe 8 – Grilled Aubergine with Tomato, Ricotta and Pesto

Not only is this a very simple recipe to prepare but also to cook. Yet the wonderful flavors really do make a lovely main course or side dish to serve not only to guests who are vegetarians but to those who love eating meat as well.

Ingredients

2 Aubergines Cut Lengthwise And Sliced Into 1 Inch Thick Pieces
5 Tablespoons Extra Virgin Olive Oil
2 Plum Tomatoes Roughly Chopped
150grams Ricotta Cheese Crumbled
3 Tablespoons Pesto (Fresh Is Best)

Instructions

1. Take the slices of aubergine and place on a baking tray before then brushing both sides with 2 to 3 tablespoons of the olive oil and then season with salt.

2. As for the tomatoes place the chopped pieces into a bowl and drizzle over them a tablespoon of olive oil and over this place the crumbled ricotta. Now set to one side (place in the refrigerator whilst you are cooking the aubergine).

3. Take the 3 tablespoons of pesto and place in a small bowl and mix into these the final olive oil and leave to one side ready to use when you serve up the aubergine, tomatoes and ricotta cheese.

4. Cook the aubergine on the barbecue over a low heat and cook on each side for 4 to 5 minutes until they have become softened. Lay the slices of aubergine on a clean plate then scatter over the top the chopped tomatoes and crumbled ricotta before then drizzling the pesto dressing over the top. Then serve to your guests.

Recipe 9 – Grilled Balsamic Mushrooms with Gorgonzola

The Gorgonzola complements the Portobello mushrooms extremely well because of their quite meaty texture.

Ingredients

6 Large or 12 Small Portobello Mushrooms
4 Tablespoons Balsamic Vinegar
2 Tablespoons Fresh Mint Chopped
2 Garlic Cloves Chopped
100grams Gorgonzola Crumbled
5 Tablespoons Olive Oil
Handful Radicchio Shredded
6 Slices French Stick

Instructions

1. Whilst the barbecue is heating up remove the stems from the Portobello mushrooms then score a criss cross pattern lightly across the tops of the mushrooms. Then place in a shallow baking dish.

2. Now in a small bowl mix together the balsamic vinegar, olive oil, mint and garlic and season with some salt and pepper. Once all these ingredients are mixed well together pour over the mushrooms remembering to turn the mushrooms over so that they are completely coated in the sauce then cover and leave to one side for 5 to 10 minutes.

3. Next take the mushrooms out of the marinade and place on the barbecue and cook on each side for 2 to 3 minutes. During the last few minutes of cooking place the slices of bread on the barbecue and toast, turn them over after about 30 seconds. When you turn the mushrooms over take the cheese and divide it equally between the mushrooms and leave on barbecue whilst you prepare the bread. By grilling the bread of the barbecue it helps to give the food a smokier flavor.

4. Take the bread and sprinkle over each piece some of the radicchio. Then top with one big mushroom or two small ones and spoon over the top any marinade left over. Serve immediately to your guests.

Recipe 10 – Halloumi & Mushroom Skewers

If you find yourself faced with guests who are vegetarians that you didn't know were coming to your barbecue then this is a really great recipe to use to make something they should enjoy.

Ingredients

250grams Halloumi Cheese
250grams Button Mushrooms
12 Rosemary Twigs Stripped Of Leaves Except The Tip
2 Tablespoons Olive Oil
2 Lemons
Small Pack Of Fresh Parsley Roughly Chopped

12 Wooden Skewers Soaked In Water For 30 Minutes

Instructions

1. Whilst the barbecue is heating up cut the Halloumi into chunks of a similar size to the mushrooms. Now take one of the rosemary twigs and one of the skewers and thread these through the cheese and mushrooms side by side. Not only will this help to make the kebabs more stable when cooking but will cause some of the rosemary flavor to be absorbed by the ingredients.

Do this for all 12 skewers and until all the mushrooms and cheese has been used up. Once the skewers are made sprinkle over some freshly ground black pepper and drizzle over some olive oil. Then set to one side ready to cook on the barbecue later.

2. Now take the lemons and zest them before then cutting them in half. Into a bowl place the lemon zest, chopped parsley and some lemon juice. Toss gently until all have been combined together well and set to one side.

3. When it comes to cooking the kebabs simply place them on to the lightly oiled barbecue grill and turn two or three times and cook for 5 to 10 minutes. As for lemon halves place these on to the barbecue cut side down and char.

4. To serve place the kebabs on a plate then take the charred lemons and squeeze them so the juice drizzles over the kebabs then sprinkle over the top of these the parsley mixture.

Recipe 11 – Hot Dressed Sweet Potato, Fennel & Feta Parcels

Again another recipe that allows you to make something special for vegetarian guests whilst also cooking what your meat eating guests will enjoy.

Ingredients

1 Sweet Potato Peeled And Cut Into Wedges
½ Small Fennel Bulb Sliced
3 Tablespoons Orange Juice Plus Zest
1 Tablespoon Olive Oil
2 Teaspoons Red Wine Vinegar
1 Teaspoon Runny Honey
1 Tablespoon Fresh Flat Leaf Parsley Chopped
1 Tablespoon Roughly Chopped Walnuts
50grams Feta Cheese Crumbled (Or You could Use Any Soft Salty Vegetarian Cheese In Place Of The Feta)

Instructions

1. Take two pieces of aluminum foil measuring 30cm and place one on top of the other. Then into the middle place the sweet potato wedges and the sliced fennel and pour over them 1 tablespoon of orange juice and 1 teaspoon of oil.

2. Now bring up the sides of the foil around the vegetables to make a bowl shape and then scrunch the edges together at the top to seal the parcel. Place the foil parcel on to the hottest part of the ready heated barbecue and cook for 35 to 45 minutes or until the potatoes inside are soft. To test the potatoes you will need to

slightly unwrap the parcels and pierce one of the potato wedges with the point of a knife.

3. Meanwhile whilst the parcel is cooking in a bowl combine together the last 2 tablespoons of orange juice with the red wine vinegar, honey, parsley, walnuts and orange zest. Add a little salt and pepper to taste.

4. When the potatoes are cooked remove from the barbecue and open the top of the parcel very carefully and pour in the dressing you made earlier. Then also add most of the feta and gently stir everything together before then scattering the rest of the feta over the top. The heat from the vegetables inside the parcel will not only bring out the flavors of the dressing but also help to warm the cheese through.

Recipe 12 – Grilled Halloumi

Although Halloumi is wonderful with many things it is just as wonderful when served on its own.

Ingredients

225grams Halloumi Cheese
1 Lemon
1 Tablespoon Olive Oil

Instructions

1. As the barbecue is heating up remove the Halloumi from its packaging and slice in slabs each between ¼ and ½ inch thick.

2. Now take the lemon and cut this into 4 to 6 slices. The slices must not be too thin or they will stick to the barbecue grill when you cook them.

3. As soon as the barbecue has heated up brush each side of the Halloumi cheese with olive oil and the same with the lemon slices. Then place them directly on to the barbecue and cook. The lemon slices should take between 1 and 2 minutes to cook whilst the

cheese will take about 6 minutes to cook. Don't forget to turn the lemon slices and the Halloumi over half way through cooking.

4. As soon as everything is cooked place the cheese on a plate and squeeze the juice out of a couple of the lemon slices before placing the remaining slices as garnish on the plate. Then serve to your guests.

Recipe 13 – Grilled Zucchini Rolls with Herbs and Cheese

This is a very inventive way of serving something that looks a little staid to your guests.

Ingredients

3 Zucchini Sliced Lengthwise Then Cut Into ¼ Inch Slices
1 Tablespoon Olive Oil
1/8 Teaspoon Salt
Pinch Freshly Ground Black Pepper
40grams Reduced Fat Soft Goat's Cheese
1 Tablespoon Fresh Parsley Leaves Minced
½ Teaspoon Lemon Juice
470grams Baby Spinach Leaves
80grams Basil Leaves

Instructions

1. After slicing up the zucchini discard the outermost ones and then brush the rest of them with olive oil on both sides. Then season with some salt and pepper. Then place on the preheated barbecue for around 4 minutes on each side or until the slices are tender.

2. Whilst the zucchini slices are cooking in a small bowl put the goat's cheese, parsley and lemon juice and mash together with fork to form a kind of cream.

3. After removing the slices of zucchini from the barbecue place ½ teaspoon of the cheese mixture about ½ inch from the end of each slice of zucchini. Then top with a few spinach leaves and a small basil leaf. Then roll up in and place them seam side down on a

plate. Once all the zucchini slices have been rolled up serve to your guests.

Recipe 14 – Cheese Stuffed Grilled Peppers

These cheese stuffed grilled peppers not only are great as a main course but as a side order to anything else you are offering to your guests.

Ingredients

4 Anaheim, Cubanella Or Baby Bell Peppers
4 Small Poblano Chillis
240grams Ricotta Cheese
240grams Cream Cheese (At Room Temperature)
120grams Fresh Parmigianino Reggiano Cheese Grated
Salt And Freshly Ground Black Pepper To Taste
Extra Virgin Olive Oil For Rubbing

Instructions

1. Into a medium bowl place the ricotta cheese along with the cream cheese and the grated Parmigianino Reggiano and mix well until they are combined together fully. Do not forget to add some salt and pepper to taste.

2. Now using a small sharp knife remove the top of the peppers with the stems and place to one side for use later. Now using the same knife cut around inside the peppers to remove the seeds.

3. Once this is done fill each one with the cheese mixture and place the tops of the peppers back in place. Then secure in place with some string. Then rub each pepper all over with the olive oil before then placing on the barbecue to cook.

4. The peppers should remain on the barbecue for at least 7 minutes and make sure that you turn them over occasionally so the skin becomes blistered but not burnt. Once the peppers are cooked transfer to a clean plate and serve to your guests. As your guests cut into the peppers the cheese mixture should start to ooze out.

NB: If you make these the night before remembering to bring them up to room temperature before you place them on the barbecue.

Recipe 15 – Fresh Herb and Goat Cheese Stuffed Grilled Portobello Mushrooms

The herbs and goat cheese help to make the meaty texture of the Portobello mushrooms a little less noticeable.

Ingredients

5 Large Portobello Mushrooms Stems Removed
220grams Fresh Goat Cheese
1 Small Garlic Clove Minced
2 Sprigs Fresh Thyme
2 Sprigs Fresh Cilantro
1 Sprig Fresh Rosemary
1 Sprig Fresh Dill
3 to 4 Large Fresh Basil Leaves
Extra Virgin Olive Oil
Salt And Freshly Ground Black Pepper To Taste

Instructions

1. After removing the stems from the mushrooms clean the dark gills before then drizzling olive oil all over them and seasoning with some salt and pepper. Then place them on the preheated barbecue face down and turn them over aver a few minutes and carry on cooking.

2. Whilst the mushrooms are cooking on the barbecue in a bowl place the goat's cheese, minced garlic and some salt and pepper to taste and combine well together. Then to this add the fresh herbs that you have torn by hand. Mix again until all the ingredients are well combined and it is a nice creamy texture.

3. As soon as the mushrooms begin to soften and a little juice escapes from then place a nice spoonful of the cream mixture into the very center of the mushroom and then close the lid of the barbecue. Cook until the cheese starts to bubble and the

Samantha Michaels

Portobello mushroom are nice and soft. Then serve immediately to your guests.

Chapter 4 – Fish Barbecue Recipes

Recipe 1 – Marinated Grilled Shrimp

A very simple but also very tasty dish and one that all your guests will enjoy even the vegetarians.

Ingredients

900grams Fresh Shrimps Peeled And Deveined
3 Garlic Cloves Minced
80ml Olive Oil
60ml Tomato Sauce
2 Tablespoons Red Wine Vinegar
2 Tablespoons Fresh Basil Chopped
½ Teaspoon Salt
¼ Teaspoon Cayenne Pepper

Wooden Skewers Soaked In Water For 30 Minutes

Instructions

1. In a large bowl place the garlic, olive oil, tomato sauce and red wine vinegar then whisk well. To this then add some salt and pepper, the chopped basil and cayenne pepper. Then to this add the shrimps. Stir everything well to make sure that the shrimps are well coated in the sauce.

2. Now cover the bowl over and place in the refrigerator for 30 minutes to an hour. Whilst the shrimps are in the refrigerator make sure that you return and stir the mixture a couple of times.

3. Whilst the shrimps are marinating you can get the barbecue going. Place the grill 6 inches above the heat source, as you will want to cook the shrimps on a medium heat.

4. After removing the shrimps from the refrigerator thread them on to the skewers piercing each one through the tail and near the head. Any left over marinade can now be discarded.

5. Just before you place the shrimps on the barbecue lightly oil the grill. Cook the shrimps on each side for 2 to 3 minutes or they become opaque in color. Then transfer to a clean plate and serve to your guests either as a starter or as a main course with some rice or couscous.

Recipe 2 – Pepper Honey Cedar Plank Salmon

The soaked cedar planks help to give the salmon a much more smoky flavor.

Ingredients

6 x 170gram Skinless And Boneless Salmon Fillets
Salt And Freshly Ground Black Pepper To Taste
Marinade
60ml Pineapple Juice
80ml Soy Sauce
2 Tablespoons White Vinegar
2 Tablespoons Lemon Juice
1 Tablespoon Olive Oil
80ml Honey
60grams Packed Brown Sugar
1 Teaspoon Ground Black Pepper
½ Teaspoon Cayenne Pepper
½ Teaspoon Paprika
¼ Teaspoon Garlic Powder
2 x 12 inch Untreated Cedar Planks

Instructions

1. Take the untreated cedar planks and place in some warm water for 1 to 2 hours.

2. In a saucepan place the pineapple juice, soy sauce, vinegar, lemon juice, olive oil and honey and warm up over a medium heat until it starts to simmer then turn the heat down slightly. Now stir in the sugar, black pepper, cayenne pepper, paprika and garlic powder and allow it to simmer for a about 15 minutes or until the mixture has reduced and is of syrupy consistency. Take off the heat and set to one side.

3. Now preheat the barbecue to a medium heat and place the planks of cedar on to the grate. You should only place the salmon on to the barbecue when the wood begins to smoke and starts to crackle a little.

4. Before you place the salmon on the barbecue grill sprinkle with some salt and pepper. The salmon should be placed directly on the planks of cedar and the lid should then be closed and remain closed for 10 minutes.

5. Open the barbecue lid after 10 minutes and place a small amount of the sauce over each salmon fillet and cook them for a further 5 minutes or until the center of the salmon has gone opaque. Serve to your guests with a crisp green salad and some of the remaining sauce poured over the top.

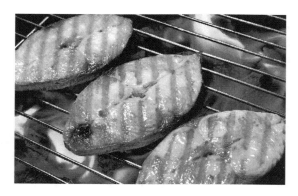

Recipe 3 – Grilled Cod

The Cajun seasoning helps to enhance the flavor and texture of this fish even more.

Ingredients

2 x 225gram Cod Fillets Cut In Half
1 Tablespoon Cajun Seasoning
½ Teaspoon Lemon Pepper
¼ Teaspoon Salt
¼ Teaspoon Freshly Ground Black Pepper
2 Tablespoons Butter
1 Lemon Juiced

2 Tablespoons Chopped Green Onions (White Part Only)

Instructions

1. Whilst the barbecue is heating up take the cod fillets and season both sides with the Cajun seasoning, lemon pepper, salt and black pepper. Then place on a plate and put to one side for now.

2. Now into a small saucepan place the butter and heat over a medium heat before then stirring in the lemon juice and the green onions and cook for about 3 minutes or until the onions are soft.

3. By now the barbecue should have heated up so place the cod fillets on to the grill, which has been lightly oiled first, and cook on each side for about 3 minutes. Whilst cooking the cod on the barbecue make sure that you baste them frequently with the butter mixture. Remove from barbecue when the cod has a golden brown color to it and flakes easily with a fork. Leave the fillets of cod to rest on a clean plate for 5 minutes before then serving to your guests.

Recipe 4 – Sweet And Spicy Seafood Kebabs

Both the scallops and shrimps absorb a great deal of the sweetness and spiciness of the marinade used. Best served with some freshly made rice and grilled pineapple rings.

Ingredients

680grams Sea Scallops
450grams Shrimps Shelled And Deveined

Marinade

½ Pineapple Crushed
80ml Chilli Sauce
2 Tablespoons Tomato Ketchup
2 Garlic Cloves Minced
2 Tablespoons Honey
1 Tablespoon Oil (Vegetable Or Canola Will Suffice)
Salt To Taste

Wooden Skewers Soaked In Water For 30 Minutes

Instructions

1. Whilst the barbecue is heating up in to a bowl combine all the marinade ingredients and stir well. Then to this add the shrimps and scallops and leave to marinate in the sauce for 10 to 15 minutes.

2. Next take the shrimps and scallops out of the marinade and thread on to the skewers alternately. Any leftover marinade should be kept for use later on.

3. Now place the kebabs on to the grill and cook on each side for 3 to 4 minutes. Whilst the kebabs are cooking brush frequently with the remaining marinade. Serve to your guests with the fresh rice and grilled pineapple when the shrimps and scallops have gone opaque.

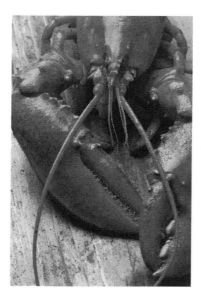

Recipe 5 – Lobster Salad with Avocado and Papaya

As soon as the lobsters are cooked add them to the salad made up of avocado, papaya, tomatoes and baby greens.

Samantha Michaels

Ingredients

4 x 800gram Live Lobsters
9 Tablespoons Olive Oil
120ml Orange Juice
3 Tablespoons Fresh Lime Juice
1 Tablespoon Seeded Minced Jalapeno Chilli
1 Tablespoon Finely Grated Lime Peel
1 ½ Teaspoons Finely Grated Orange Peel
2 Avocados Halved, Pitted, Peeled And Cut Into ½ Inch Pieces
4 Medium Tomatoes Seeded And Cut Into ½ Inch Pieces
1 Large Papaya Peeled, Seeded And Cut Into ½ Inch Pieces
2Kg Mixed Baby Greens

470grams Mesquite Smoke Chips Soaked In Water For 30 Minutes Then Drained

Instructions

1. Bring a large pan of boiling salt water to the boil and then drop the lobster's head first into it. Cover the pan over and boil the lobsters for 2 minutes. Remove from water and transfer to a chopping board and immediately split the lobsters open lengthwise using a heavy knife and crack the claws.

2. Now place the lobsters cut side up on to the preheated barbecue and cover then grill for 6 minutes. Turn the lobsters over and grill until just cooked through about another 5 minutes. Then remove from the barbecue and remove the meat from the shells and cut into ½ inch pieces and place in a large bowl.

3. In a medium size whisk together the oil, orange juice, lime juice, minced jalapeno chilli, lime peel and orange peel and add a little salt and pepper to taste. If you would prefer you could actually make this dressing the day before.

4. Next take the pieces of avocado, tomatoes and papaya and place them in a bowl along with the lobster and pour over about 120ml of the dressing you made earlier again add a little salt and pepper to taste.

5. In another bowl toss the baby greens with the rest of the dressing you made earlier and then divide it equally among plates and on top place some of the lobster mixture and serve to your guests.

Recipe 6 – Shrimp and Broccoli Packets

This is a great recipe to use if you want to offer this as a main to your vegetarian guests whilst serving steaks to the rest.

Ingredients

225grams Medium Size Fresh Shrimps Peeled And Deveined
240grams Instant Rice
2 Teaspoons Seafood Seasoning
2 Garlic Cloves Minced And Divided
480grams Broccoli Florets
30grams Butter Cut Into Pieces
8 Ice Cubes
120ml Water

2 Sheets Of Aluminum Foil Measuring 12 x 18 Inches

Instructions

1. Preheat the barbecue making sure that the lid is closed so the temperature inside reaches 450 degrees Fahrenheit. Place the barbecue grill around 5 inches above the heat source as you will want to cook these packets on a medium to high heat.

2. In the center of the aluminum foil (dull side facing you) place half of the shrimps. Then around them place some of the rice as well as sprinkling some over the top of the shrimps. Also add a teaspoon of the seafood seasoning and a quarter of the garlic on top. Then place some of the broccoli on top of the shrimps before then adding another ¼ of the garlic and 15 grams of butter.

On top of all these place 4 ice cubes and bring the sides of the foil up and double fold the top and one end. Through the open end then pour 60ml of water before then sealing this end up.

Don't fold the packets too tightly as there needs to be space in side them for the heat to circulate. Do this for the same for the second packet.

4. Now place the packets on to the grill and close the lid then cook the packets for between 9 and 13 minutes. Just before serving open the packets up and stir the rice and then place on clean plates.

Recipe 7 – Fruity Seafood Kebabs

These kebabs are loaded with lots of wonderful fruity flavors and need to be good on a very high heat very quickly. As soon as the shark is cooked to your likely remove them from the grill.

Ingredients

450grams Shark
450grams Large Shrimps Peeled And Deveined
450grams Large Scallops
1 Pineapple Peeled And Cored
2 Peaches Peeled And Seeded
4 Semi Green Bananas Peeled
12 Large Strawberries Capped
2 Apples Cored And Quartered

Instructions

1. Cut the fruit and shark into cuts that fit on to a kebab skewer. Once done then thread alternate pieces of fruit, shark, scallop and shrimp on to each skewer.

2. Once all kebabs are ready place them onto the lightly oiled barbecue grill, which is set 4 inches above the heat source and cook for 10 minutes. Remember to turn them half way through the cooking time and then serve immediately to your guests with some fresh green salad or with some couscous or rice.

Recipe 8 – Trout with Lime and Thyme

The use of lime and thyme helps to enhance the flavor of this very oily fish even more.

Ingredients

2 x 115gram Trout Fillets
Juice Of 1 Lime
1 Tablespoon Olive Oil
1 Tablespoon Fresh Thyme Minced
2 Garlic Cloves Minced
½ Teaspoon Coarsely Ground Black Pepper
1/8 Teaspoon Cayenne Pepper (You Can Add More If You Wish If You Cannot Really Taste It)

Instructions

1. In a bowl mix together the lime juice, olive oil; thyme, garlic, black pepper and cayenne pepper then pour it into a resealable bag.

2. Now place the trout fillets in the same bag seal and turn over several times gently to ensure that the fillets are well coated in the mixture. Place in the refrigerator for at least 30 minutes to allow the trout fillets to absorb as much of the marinade as possible. If possible leave the fish in the marinade as long as possible as more of the marinades flavors will then be absorbed by it.

3. Preheat the barbecue placing the grill 6 inches above the heat source because you will want to cook the trout fillets on a medium heat.

4. After removing the trout from the bag before placing on the barbecue lightly oil the grill. Make sure that you shake any excess marinade off the fish before placing and the grill and any left in the bag can now be discarded.

5. Cook the trout fillets on the barbecue for between 10 to 15 minutes or until the flesh of the fish flakes easily. Make sure that you turn the fish over once whilst cooking. Once cooked place on a

clean plate and serve with some rice or baby new potatoes and a crisp green salad.

Recipe 9 – Grilled Oysters

When cooking these oysters you need to watch them very carefully. As soon as the shells begin to open remove them from the barbecue and serve. Not only great as a main course but also a starter.

Ingredients

12 Oysters Per Person
Salt And Freshly Ground Black Pepper
Butter Melted
Hot Pepper Sauce
Worcestershire Sauce
Lemon Wedges

Instructions

1. Whilst the barbecue is heating up clean the oyster shells making sure that all mud is removed from them.

2. Once the barbecue has heated place the unopened oysters on to the grill and close the lid. Cook until the shells start to open this should take around 6 minutes then remove from the grill.

3. Now open the oysters up further and cut them away from the shell. Place on a plate a serve to your guests along with the sauces and seasonings mentioned above. However before you do serve drizzle some melted butter over them.

NB: Make sure that you grill the oysters in batches as this will help to ensure that everyone who wants oysters will have hot ones.

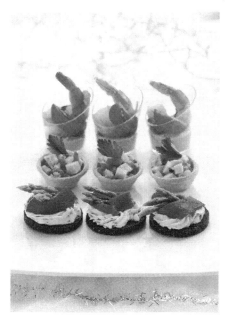

Recipe 10 – Sweet and Spicy Grilled Shrimp

The sweet and spicy marinade in which these shrimps are left helps to bring out the subtle flavor of the shrimps even more.

Ingredients

450grams Medium Sized Shrimps Peeled And Deveined
120ml Chilli Garlic Sauce
120ml Honey

6 Bamboo Skewers Soaked In Water For 20 Minutes

Instructions

1. Whilst the barbecue is heating up in a small bowl mix together the honey and chilli garlic sauce. Make sure that you place the grill of the barbecue 6 inches above the heat source, as you will want to cook the shrimps on a medium heat.

2. Remove the skewers from the water and then thread on to these the shrimps piercing them both through head and tails. Then place on the barbecue and baste with the sauce. Turn the shrimps

regularly and baste each time you turn them and cook for around 10 minutes or until the shrimps have all turned pink and feel firm to the touch.

3. Now place the kebabs on to a clean plate and drizzle over any remaining sauce and serve alongside some rice or fresh crispy bread.

Recipe 11 – Honey Ginger Grilled Salmon

The honey and ginger help to enhance the flavor of the salmon a great deal.

Ingredients

680grams Salmon Fillets
1 Teaspoon Ground Ginger
1 Teaspoon Garlic Powder
80ml Reduced Sodium Soy Sauce
80ml Orange Juice
60ml Honey
1 Green Onion Chopped

Instructions

1. In a large resealable bag place the ground ginger, garlic powder, soy sauce, orange juice, honey and green onions. Close the bag and shake vigorously to ensure that the entire ingredients are combined well together.

2. Open the bag and into this place the salmon fillet and tightly seal the bag closed. Now gently turn the bag over several times to help coat the fillet evenly in the marinade before then placing it in the refrigerator for between 15 and 30 minutes. The longer you leave the salmon in the marinade the more of the sauces flavors will be absorbed by the fish. During this time also turn the bag over occasionally.

3. As soon as the barbecue is heated up lightly oil the grill and place the salmon on to it. Do not throw any remaining marinade away as you will use this to baste the fish whilst it is cooking.

4. Cook the fish for between 12 and 15 minutes depending on how thick the fillet is or until it flakes easily with a fork. Then serve immediately with a crisp green salad, boiled new potatoes and some crusty bread.

Recipe 12 – Fresh Citrus Salmon

Salmon is quite an oily fish and the lemon, lime and orange help to counteract some of this.

Ingredients

4 Salmon Fillets With Skin On
2 Small Lemons
2 Medium Oranges
1 Large Lime
100ml Freshly Squeezed Lemon Juice
100ml Freshly Squeezed Orange Juice
50ml Freshly Squeezed Lime Juice
100grams Mixed Leaf Lettuce
250grams Cherry Tomatoes Halved
2 Large Garlic Cloves Divided
4 Tablespoons Balsamic Vinegar Divided
2 Teaspoons Fresh Dill Chopped
Olive Oil
Sea Salt And Freshly Ground Black Pepper To Taste

Instructions

1. Thoroughly wash the salmon fillets then pat dry with some paper towels. Once the fillets are dry drizzle over some olive oil and grind some salt and pepper on to the skin side and rub in. Place on a plate, cover and place in the refrigerator for 30 minutes.

2. After peeling the oranges, lemons and lime separate up the segments. Make sure that you retain any juices and mix these segments of fruit in a bowl with a little olive oil, ½ crushed garlic clove and refrigerate.

3. Next into a bowl combine together the dill, 1 crushed garlic clove, the lime, lemon and orange juice and drizzle in a little olive oil. Also sprinkle in a little salt and pepper.

4. Now remove the salmon from the fridge and place in a shallow baking dish or resealable bag and cover with the dill marinade. Place back in the refrigerator and leave there for a further 2 hours.

5. 20 minutes before you intend to start cooking the salmon on the preheated barbecue remove from the fridge. During this time you can make the salad to go with the salmon. To make the salad place the segments of lemon, lime and orange in a bowl with the tomato halve and the salad leaves and drizzle over it all a tablespoon of balsamic vinegar before then tossing everything very lightly.

6. After rubbing the grate very lightly with a clove of garlic place the salmon fillets skin side down and cover with a very big well vented saucepan lid and leave. Allow remaining under this lid for 2 minutes before then turning the fillets over remembering to replace the lid over the top and cook for a further two minutes.

Once the salmon is cooked remove from heat and place a small amount of the salad mix (keeping back any citrus segments) and place the fillets of salmon on top skin side up. Garnish then with the citrus segments and some of the cherry tomato halves and also drizzle some balsamic vinegar over the top then serve.

Recipe 13 – Barbecued Marinated Swordfish

You will find that swordfish has quite a meaty texture and often needs to be cooked on a medium heat for a little longer than other types of fish do.

Ingredients

4 Swordfish Steaks
4 Garlic Cloves Minced
75ml White Wine
4 Tablespoons Lemon Juice
2 Tablespoons Soy Sauce
2 Tablespoons Olive Oil

1 Tablespoon Savory Seasoning
¼ Teaspoon Salt
1/8 Teaspoon Freshly Ground Black Pepper
1 Tablespoon Fresh Parsley Chopped (Garnish Optional)
4 Lemon Slices (Garnish Optional)

Instructions

1. In a bowl whisk together the garlic, white wine, lemon juice, soy sauce, olive oil, savory seasoning, salt and pepper. Then pour over the swordfish steaks, which have been placed in a shallow baking dish. Remember to turn the steaks over to ensure that they are well coated in the sauce then place in the refrigerator for 1 hour. Whilst the steaks are marinating turn them over frequently.

2. Whilst the barbecue is heating up remove the swordfish steaks from the refrigerator so that they can be cooked at room temperature. Also before placing the steaks on the barbecue brush the grill with oil which is placed 4 inches above the heat source as these will need cooking on a very high heat.

3. After placing the swordfish steaks on the barbecue cook for 6 to 6 minutes on each side then serve garnished with the parsley and lemon wedges to your guests on clean plates with some green beans and new potatoes.

Recipe 14 – Barbecued Stuffed Red Snapper

If you are not able to get red snapper then use mullet instead.

Ingredients

6 x 100gram Red Snapper (Mullet) Fillets
110grams Cooked Prawns
110grams Cooked Crab Meat
2 Tablespoons Butter
5 Tablespoons Fresh Breadcrumbs
1 Tablespoon Butter
1 Spring Onion Chopped
1 Stalk Celery Diced
1 Garlic Clove Minced

1 Tablespoon Fresh Parsley Chopped
1/8 Teaspoon Salt
1/8 Teaspoon Freshly Ground Black Pepper

Instructions

1. To make the stuffing for the fish melt 2 tablespoons of butter in a frying pan then add to this the fresh breadcrumbs and sauté over a medium heat until the breadcrumbs have gone brown. Remove from heat and place the breadcrumbs in a bowl.

2. Now add a further tablespoon of butter to the frying pan and to this add the spring onions, celery and garlic and cook until all are tender then add these to the breadcrumbs then stir in both the prawns and crab meat, the parsley and some salt and pepper. Then toss gently.

3. Take eight large pieces of aluminum foil and on two sheets place one of the fish fillets then mound the stuffing on top of the fish. Now curl up the sides of the foil so that each one forms a tray and place on the barbecue grill and close the lid and cook the fish for between 20 and 25 minutes or until the fish flakes easily with a fork.

4. Once the fish is cooked remove from aluminum foil and place on plates with some fresh green salad and some crusty bread. Then serve to your guests.

Recipe 15 – Barbecued Tuna with Honey Glaze

The honey glaze helps to enhance the smoky flavors of the tuna when cooked on the barbecue.

Ingredients

450gram Tuna Fillets
4 Tablespoons Olive Oil
4 Tablespoons Lime Juice
2 Tablespoons Balsamic Vinegar
2 Garlic Cloves Minced
1 Tablespoon Fresh Ginger Root Peeled And Minced

Small Bunch Fresh Coriander Chopped

Honey Glaze

4 Tablespoons Honey
2 Tablespoons Olive Oil
2 Tablespoons Fresh Coriander Finely Chopped

Instructions

1. In a medium size bowl mix together the olive oil, lime juice, balsamic vinegar, garlic, ginger and coriander. Then add to this the tuna fillets, which you turn over several times to ensure that they are evenly coated in the marinade. Cover the bowl over and leave in the refrigerator to marinate for several hours.

2. Preheat the barbecue to cook the fish on a high heat and whilst the barbecue is heating up prepare the honey glaze. To make the glaze simply place the honey, olive oil and coriander in a small bowl and whisk. Once all these ingredients are combined put the bowl to one side ready for use later.

3. Once the barbecue has heated up place the tuna fillets on to the lightly oiled grill and close the lid. Cook the tuna with the lid closed for 1 to 2 minutes then flip them fillets over and cook for a further 1 to 2 minutes with the lid closed. Now open the lid and continue to cook the tuna fillets until they are barely done, making sure that you baste them frequently with any leftover marinade.

4. Before the fish is cooked right through now brush both sides of the fish with the honey glaze and then remove from the barbecue. Serve with some noodles or with a nice crisp salad.

MORE 70 BEST EVER RECIPES EBOOKS REVEALED AT MY AUTHOR PAGE:-

CLICK HERE TO ACCESS THEM NOW

34878219R00050

Made in the USA
Lexington, KY
28 March 2019